Current Clinical Strategies

Critical Care Medicine

Year 2000 Edition

Matthew Brenner, MD
Associate Professor of Medicine
Pulmonary and Critical Care Division
University of California, Irvine

Michael Safani, PharmD
Assistant Clinical Professor
School of Pharmacy
University of California, San Francisco

Thomas T. Vovan, MD	*John Roper, MD*
Naeem Rana, MD	*D. Serna, MD*
Wenchao Wu, MD	*Feras Hawari, MD*
Ledford L. Powell, MD	*Kuldip Gill, MD*
Steve Marks, DO	*Ziad Tannous, MD*

Division of Pulmonary and Critical Care Medicine
College of Medicine
University of California, Irvine

Current Clinical Strategies Publishing

www.ccspublishing.com

Digital Book and Updates

Purchasers of this book may download the digital book and updates of this text at the Current Clinical Strategies Publishing internet site: www.ccspublishing.com.

Current Clinical Strategies Publishing

www.ccspublishing.com

27071 Cabot Road
Laguna Hills, California 92653
Phone: 800-331-8227
E-Mail: info@ccspublishing.com

Printed in USA   ISBN 1-881528-774

Contents

Critical Care Patient Management

Thomas Vovan, MD
Ledford L Powell, MD

Critical Care History and Physical Examination

Chief complaint: Reason for admission to the ICU and system failure responsible for admission.

History of present illness: This section should included pertinent chronological events leading up to hospitalization, and it should include events during hospitalization and eventual admission to the ICU.

Prior cardiac history: Angina (stable, unstable, changes in frequency), exacerbating factors (exertional, rest angina). History of myocardial infarction, heart failure, coronary artery bypass graft operation, angioplasty placement. Previous exercise treadmill testing, ECHO, ejection fraction. Request old EKG, ECHO, stress test results, and angiographic studies.

Chest pain characteristics:
  A. **Pain:** Quality of pain, pressure, squeezing, tightness
  B. **Onset:** Exertional, awakening from sleep, relationship to activities of daily living (ADLs), such as eating, bathing, and grooming.
  C. **Severity and quality:** Pressure, tightness, sharp, pleuritic
  D. **Radiation:** Arm, jaw, shoulder
  E. **Associated symptoms:** Diaphoresis, dyspnea, back pain, GI symptoms.
  F. **Duration:** Minutes, hours, days.
  G. **Relieving factors:** Nitroclycerine, rest.

Cardiac risk factors: Age, male, diabetes, hypercholesteremia, Low HDL, hypertension, smoking, previous coronary artery disease, family history of arteriosclerosis (eg, myocardial infarction in males less than 50 years old, stroke)

Congestive heart failure symptoms: Orthopnea (number of pillows), paroxysmal nocturnal dyspnea, dyspnea on exertional, edema.

Peripheral vascular disease symptoms: Claudication, transient ischemic attack, cerebral vascular accident.

COPD exacerbation symptoms: Shortness of breath, fever, chills, wheezing, sputum production, hemoptysis (quantify), corticosteroid use, previous intubation.

Past medical history: Peptic ulcer disease, renal disease, diabetes, COPD. Functional status prior to hospitalization.

Medications: Dose and frequency. Use of nitroglycerine, beta-agonist, steroids.

Social history: Tobacco use, alcohol consumption, HIV risk factors, intravenous drug use.

Allergies: Penicillins, contrast dye, aspirin; describe the specific reaction (eg, anaphylaxis, wheezing, rash, hypotension)

Review of systems: Review symptoms related to each organ system.

Critical Care Physical Examination

Vital signs:

Temperature, pulse, respiratory rate, BP (vital signs should be given in ranges)

Input/Output: Urine

Special parameters: Arterial blood gasses, pulmonary artery wedge pressure (PAWP), systemic vascular resistance (SVR), ventilator settings.

General: Mental status, Glasgow coma score, degree of distress.

HEENT: PERRLA, EOMI.

Lungs: Inspection, percussion, auscultation for wheezes, crackles, rubs.

Cardiac: Regular rate and rhythm.

Cardiac murmurs: 1/6 = faint; 2/6 = clear; 3/6 - loud; 4/6 = palpable; 5/6 = heard with stethoscope off the chest; 6/6 = heard without stethoscope.

Abdomen: Bowel sounds normoactive, abdomen soft and nontender.

Extremities: Cyanosis, clubbing, edema, peripheral pulses 2+.

Skin: Capillary refill and skin turgor.

Neuro

Deficits in strength, sensation.

Deep tendon reflexes: 0 = absent; 1 = diminished; 2 = normal; 3 = brisk; 4 = hyperactive clonus.

Motor Strength: 0 = no contractility; 1 = contractility but no joint motion; 2 = motion without gravity; 3 = motion against gravity; 4 = some resistance; 5 = motion against full resistance (normal).

Labs: CBC, INR/PTT; Chem 7, chem 12, Mg, pH/pCO2/pO2. CXR, EKG, other diagnostic studies.

Impression/Problem list: Discuss diagnosis and plan for each problem by system.

Neurologic Problems: List and discuss neurologic problems

Pulmonary Problems: Ventilator management, DVT prophylaxis.

Cardiac Problems: Arrhythmia, chest pain, angina

GI Problems: H2 blockers, nasogastric tubes, nutrition.

Genitourinary and Electrolytes Problems: Fluid status: IV fluids, electrolyte therapy.

Hematologic Problems: Blood or blood products

Infectious Disease: Plans for antibiotic therapy; antibiotic day number, culture results.

Endocrine/Nutrition: Serum glucose control, parenteral or enteral nutrition, diet.

Admission Check List

1. **Call and request** old chart, EKG, and X-rays.
2. **Stat labs:** CBC, Chem 7, INR, PTT, C&S, ABG, UA.
3. **Labs:** Toxicology screens and drug levels.
4. **Cultures:** Blood culture x 2, urine and sputum culture (before initiating antibiotics), sputum Gram stain, urinalysis.
5. **CXR, EKG**, diagnostic studies.
6. **Discuss case with resident, attending**, and family.

Critical Care Progress Note

ICU Day Number:
Antibiotic Day Number:
Subjective: Patient is awake and alert. Note any events that occurred overnight.
Objective: Temperature, maximum, temperature, pulse, respiratory rate, BP, 24 hr input and output, pulmonary artery
pressure, pulmonary capillary wedge pressure, cardiac output.
Lungs: Clear bilaterally
Cardiac: Regular rate and rhythm, no murmur, no rubs.
Abdomen: Bowel sounds normoactive, soft-nontender.
Neuro: No local deficits in strength, sensation.
Extremities: No cyanosis, clubbing, edema, peripheral pulses 2+.
Labs: CBC, ABG, Chem 7.
EKG: CXR:
Impression and Plan: Give an overall impression, and then discuss impression and plan by organ system:
    Cardiovascular:
    Pulmonary:
    Neurological:
    Gastrointestinal:
    Infectious:
    Endocrine:
    Nutrition:

Procedure Note

A procedure note should be written in the chart when a procedure is performed. Procedure notes are brief operative notes.

Procedure Note

Date and time:
Procedure:
Indications:
Patient Consent: Document that the indications, risks and alternatives to the procedure were explained to the patient. Note that the patient was given the opportunity to ask questions and that the patient consented to the procedure in writing.
Lab tests: Relevant labs, such as the INR and CBC
Anesthesia: Local with 2% lidocaine
Description of Procedure: Briefly describe the procedure, including sterile prep, anesthesia method, patient position, devices used, anatomic location of procedure, and outcome.
Complications and Estimated Blood Loss (EBL):
Disposition: Describe how the patient tolerated the procedure.
Specimens: Describe any specimens obtained and labs tests which were ordered.

Discharge Note

The discharge note should be written in the patient's chart prior to discharge.

Discharge Note

Date/time:
Diagnoses:
Treatment: Briefly describe therapy provided during hospitalization, including antibiotic therapy, surgery, and cardiovascular drugs.
Studies Performed: Electrocardiograms, CT scan.
Discharge medications:
Follow-up Arrangements:

Fluids and Electrolytes

Maintenance Fluids Guidelines:
   70 kg Adult: D5 1/4 NS with 20 mEq KCl/Liter at 125 mL/hr.
Specific Replacement Fluids for Specific Losses:
   Gastric (nasogastric tube, emesis): D5 ½ NS with 20 mEq/Liter KCL.
   Diarrhea: D5LR with 15 mEq/liter KCl. Provide 1 liter of replacement for each 1 kg or 2.2 lb of body weight lost.
   Bile: D5LR with 25 mEq/liter (½ amp) of sodium bicarbonate.
   Pancreatic: D5LR with 50 mEq/liter (1 amp) sodium bicarbonate.

Blood Component Therapy

A. **Packed red blood cells (PRBCs).** Each unit provides 250-400 cc of volume, and each unit should raise hemoglobin by 1 gm/dL and hematocrit by 3%. PRBCs are usually requested in two unit increments.

B. **Type and screen.** Blood is tested for A, B, Rh antigens, and antibodies to donor erythrocytes. If blood products are required, the blood can be rapidly prepared by the blood bank. O negative blood is used in patients when type and screen information is not available, but the need for transfusion is emergent.

C. **Type and cross match** sets aside specific units of packed donor red blood cells. If blood is needed on an urgent basis, type and cross should be requested.

D. **Platelets.** Indicated for bleeding if there is thrombocytopenia or thrombopathy in the setting of uncontrolled bleeding. Each unit of platelet concentrate should raise the platelet count by 5,000-10,000. Platelets are usually transfused 6-10 units at a time, which should increase the platelet count by 40-60,000. Thrombocytopenia is defined as a platelet count of less than 60,000. For surgery, the count should be greater than 50,000. Thrombocytopenia has been associated with heparin, and thrombopathy has been seen with aspirin, nonsteroidal anti-inflammatory drugs (NSAIDs), dipyridamole, phenothiazines, penicillins, lidocaine, and cocaine

E. **Fresh Frozen Plasma (FFP)** is used for active bleeding secondary to liver disease, warfarin overdose, dilutional coagulopathy secondary to multiple blood transfusions, disseminated intravascular coagulopathy, vitamin K and coagulation factor deficiencies. Administration of FFP requires ABO typing, but not cross matching.
   1. Each unit contains coagulation factors in normal concentration.
   2. Two to four units are usually required for therapeutic intervention, and the frequency of dosing depends on clinical response.

F. **Cryoprecipitate**
   1. Indicated in patients with Hemophilia A, Von Willebrand's disease, and any state of hypofibrinogenemia requiring replacement (DIC), or reversal of thrombolytic therapy.
   2. Cryoprecipitate contains factor VIII, fibrinogen, and Von Willebrand factor.
   3. The goal of therapy is to maintain the fibrinogen level above 100 mL/dL. This is usually achieved with 10 units given over 3-5 minutes.

Central Parenteral Nutrition

Infuse 40-50 mL/hr of amino acid dextrose solution in the first 24 hr; increase daily by 40 mL/hr increments until providing 1.3-2 x basal energy requirement and 1.2-1.7 gm protein/kg/d (see formula, page 130)

Standard Solution per Liter

Amino acid solution (Aminosyn) 7-10%	500 mL
Dextrose 40-70%	500 mL
Sodium	35 mEq
Potassium	36 mEq
Chloride	35 mEq
Calcium	4.5 mEq
Phosphate	9 mMol
Magnesium	8.0 mEq
Acetate	82-104 mEq
Multi-Trace Element Formula	1 mL/d
Regular insulin (if indicated)	10-20 U/L
Multivitamin 12 (2 amp)	10 mL/d
Vitamin K (in solution, SQ, IM)	10 mg/week
Vitamin B 12	1000 mcg/week

Fat Emulsion:
- Intralipid 20% 500 mL/d IVPB infused in parallel with standard solution at 1 mL/min x 15 min; if no adverse reactions, increase to 20-50 mL/hr. Serum triglyceride level should be checked 6h after end of infusion (maintain <250 mg/dL).

Cyclic Total Parenteral Nutrition
- 12-hour night schedule; taper continuous infusion in morning by reducing rate to half original rate for 1 hour. Further reduce rate by half for an additional hour, then discontinue. Restart TPN in evening. Taper at beginning and end of cycle. Final rate should be 185 mL/hr for 9-10h with 2 hours of taper at each end, for total of 2000 mL.

Peripheral Parenteral Supplementation
- Amino acid solution (ProCalamine) 3% up to 3 L/d at 125 cc/h OR
- Combine 500 mL amino acid solution 7% or 10% (Aminosyn) and 500 mL 20% dextrose and electrolyte additive and infuse at up to 100 cc/hr in parallel with: Intralipid 10% or 20% at 1 mL/min for 15 min (test dose); if no adverse reactions, infuse 500 mL/d at 20 mL/hr.

Special Medications
- Cimetidine (Tagamet) 300 mg IV q6-8h or in TPN OR
- Ranitidine (Zantac) 50 mg IV q6-8h.
- Insulin sliding scale.

Labs

Baseline: Draw labs below. CXR, plain film for tube placement

Daily Labs: Chem 7, osmolality, CBC, cholesterol, triglyceride (6h after end of infusion), serum phosphate, magnesium, calcium, urine specific gravity.

Weekly Labs: Protein, iron, TIBC, INR/PTT, 24h urine nitrogen and creatinine. Pre-albumin, transferrin, albumin, total protein, AST, ALT, GGT, alkaline phosphatase, LDH, amylase, total bilirubin.

Enteral Nutrition

General Measures: Daily weights, nasoduodenal feeding tube. Head of bed at 30 degrees while enteral feeding and 2 hours after completion. Record bowel movements.

Continuous Enteral Infusion: Initial enteral solution (Osmolite, Pulmocare, Jevity) 30 mL/hr. Measure residual volume q1h x 12h, then tid; hold feeding for 1 h if residual is more than 100 mL of residual. Increase rate by 25-50 mL/hr at 24 hr intervals as tolerated until final rate of 50-100 mL/hr (1 cal/mL) as tolerated. Three tablespoons of protein powder (Promix) may be added to each 500 cc of solution. Flush tube with 100 cc water q8h.

Enteral Bolus Feeding: Give 50-100 mL of enteral solution (Osmolite, Pulmocare, Jevity) q3h initially. Increase amount in 50 mL steps to max of 250-300 mL q3-4h; 30 kcal of nonprotein calories/d and 1.5 gm protein/kg/d. Before each feeding measure residual volume, and delay feeding by 1 h if >100 mL. Flush tube with 100 cc of water after each bolus.

Special Medications:
-Metoclopramide (Reglan) 10-20 mg PO, IM, IV, or in J tube q6h.
-Cimetidine (Tagamet) 300 mg PO tid-qid or 37.5-100 mg/h IV or 300 mg IV q6-8h **OR**
-Ranitidine (Zantac) 50 mg IV q6-8h or 150 mg in J-tube bid.

Symptomatic Medications:
-Loperamide (Imodium) 24 mg PO or in J-tube q6h, max 16 mg/d prn **OR**
-Diphenoxylate/atropine (Lomotil) 5-10 mL (2.5 mg/5 mL) PO or in J-tube q4-6h, max 12 tabs/d **OR**
-Kaopectate 30 cc PO or in J-tube q6h.

Radiographic Evaluation of Common Interventions

I. Central Intravenous Lines
   A. Central venous catheters should be located well above the right atrium, and not in a neck vein. Rule out pneumothorax by checking that the lung markings extend completely to the rib cages on both sides. An upright, expiratory x-ray may be helpful. Examine for hydropericardium ("water bottle" sign, mediastinal widening).

   B. Pulmonary artery catheter tips should be located centrally and posteriorly, and not more than 3-5 cm from midline.

II. Endotracheal tubes.
Verify that the tube is located 3 cm below the vocal cords and 2-4cm above the carina; the tip of tube should be at the level of aortic arch.

III. Tracheostomies.
Verify by chest x-ray that the tube is located halfway between the stoma and the carina; the tube should be parallel to the long axis of the trachea. The tube should be approximately 2/3 of width of the trachea; the cuff should not cause bulging of the trachea walls. Check for subcutaneous air in the neck tissue and for mediastinal widening secondary to air leakage.

IV. Nasogastric tubes.
Verify that the tube is in the stomach and not coiled in the esophagus or trachea. The tip of the tube should not be near the gastroesophageal junction.

V. Chest tubes.
A chest tube for pneumothorax drainage should be superior, near the level of the third intercostal space. To drain a free flowing pleural effusion, the tube should be located inferior-posteriorly, at or about the level of the eighth intercostal space. Verify that the side port of the tube is within the thorax.

VI. Mechanical ventilation. Obtain a chest x-ray to rule out pneumothorax, subcutaneous emphysema, pneumomediastinum or subpleural air cysts. Lung infiltrates or atelectasis may diminish or disappear after initiation of mechanical ventilation because of increased aeration of the affected lung lobe.

Arterial Line Placement

Procedure
1. Obtain a 20 gauge 1 ½-2 inch catheter over needle assembly (Angiocath), arterial line setup (transducer, tubing and pressure bag containing heparinized saline), arm board, sterile dressing, lidocaine, 3 cc syringe, 25 gauge needle, 3-O silk suture.
2. The radial artery is the most frequently used artery. Use the Allen test to verify patency of the radial and ulnar arteries. Place the extremity on an arm board with a gauze roll behind the wrist to maintain hyperextension.
3. Prep the skin with povidone-iodine and drape; infiltrate 1% lidocaine using a 25-gauge needle. Choose site where the artery appears most superficial and distal.
4. Palpate the artery with the left hand, and advance the catheter-over-needle assembly into the artery at a 30-degree angle to the skin. When a flash of blood is seen, hold the needle in place and advance the catheter into the artery. Occlude the artery with manual pressure while the pressure tubing is connected.
5. Advance the guide-wire into the artery, and pass the catheter over the guide-wire.
6. Suture the catheter in place with 3-0 silk and apply dressing.

Central Venous Catheterization

I. Indications for Central Venous Catheter Cannulation: Monitoring of central venous pressures in shock or heart failure; management of fluid status; insertion of a transvenous pacemaker; administration of total parenteral nutrition; administration of vesicants (chemotherapeutic agents).

II. Location: The internal jugular approach is relatively contraindicated in patients with carotid bruits, stenosis, or aneurysm. The subclavian approach has an increased risk of pneumothorax in patients with emphysema or bullae. The external jugular or internal jugular approach is preferable in patients with coagulopathy or thrombocytopenia because of the ease of external compression for hemostasis. In patients with unilateral lung pathology or a chest tube already in place, the catheter should be placed on the side of predominant pathology or on the side with the chest tube if present.

III. Technique for Insertion of External Jugular Vein Catheter
   1. The external jugular vein extends from the angle of the mandible to behind the middle of the clavicle where it joins with the subclavian vein. Place patient in Trendelenburg's position. Cleanse skin with Betadine-iodine solution, and, using sterile technique, inject 1% lidocaine to produce a skin weal. Apply digital pressure to the external jugular vein above the clavicle to distend the vein.

2. With a 16-gauge thin wall needle, advance the needle into the vein. Then pass a J-guide wire through the needle; the wire should advance without resistance. Remove the needle, maintaining control over the guide wire at all times. Nick the skin with a No. 11 scalpel blade.
3. With the guide wire in place, pass the central catheter over the wire and remove the guide wire after the catheter is in place. Cover the catheter hub with a finger to prevent air embolization.
4. Attach a syringe to the catheter hub and ensure that there is free back-flow of dark venous blood. Attach the catheter to intravenous infusion.
5. Secure the catheter in place with 2-0 silk suture and tape. The catheter should be replaced weekly or if there is any sign of infection.
6. Obtain a CXR to confirm position and rule out pneumothorax.

IV. **Internal Jugular Vein Cannulation.** The internal jugular vein is positioned behind the stemocleidomastoid muscle lateral to the carotid artery. The catheter should be placed at a location at the upper confluence of the two bellies of the stemocleidomastoid, at the level of the cricoid cartilage.

1. Place the patient in Trendelenburg's position and turn the patient's head to the contralateral side.
2. Choose a location on the right or left. If lung function is symetrical and no chest tubes are in place, the right side is preferred because of the direct path to the superior vena cava. Prepare the skin with Betadine solution using sterile technique and a drape. Infiltrate the skin and deeper tissues with 1% lidocaine.
3. Palpate the carotid artery. Using a 22-gauge scout needle and syringe, direct the needle lateral to the carotid artery towards the ipsilateral nipple at a 30-degree angle to the neck. While aspirating, advance the needle until the vein is located and blood flows back into the syringe.
4. Remove the scout needle and advance a 16-gauge, thin wall catheter-over-needle with an attached syringe along the same path as the scout needle. When back flow of blood is noted into the syringe, advance the catheter into the vein. Remove the needle and confirm back flow of blood through the catheter and into the syringe. Remove the syringe, and use a finger to cover the catheter hub to prevent air embolization.
5. With the 16-gauge catheter in position, advance a 0.89 mm x 45 cm spring guide wire through the catheter. The guidewire should advance easily without resistance.
6. With the guidewire in position, remove the catheter and use a No. 11 scalpel blade to nick the skin.
7. Place the central vein catheter over the wire, holding the wire secure at all times. Pass the catheter into the vein, remove the guidewire, and suture the catheter with 0 silk suture, tape, and connect it to an IV infusion.
8. Obtain a chest x-ray to rule out pneumothorax and confirm position of the catheter.

V. **Subclavian Vein Cannulation**. The subclavian vein is located in the angle formed by the medial 1/3 of the clavicle and the first rib.

1. Position the patient supine with a rolled towel located between the patient's scapulae, and turn the patient's head towards the contralateral side. Prepare the area with betadine iodine solution, and, using sterile technique, drape the area and infiltrate 1% lidocaine into the skin and tissues.

2. Advance the 16-gauge catheter-over-needle, with syringe attached, into a location inferior to the mid-point of the clavicle, until the clavicle bone and needle come in contact.
3. Slowly probe down with the needle until the needle slips under the clavicle, and advance it slowly towards the vein until the catheter needle enters the vein, and a back flow of venous blood enters the syringe. Remove the syringe, and cover the catheter hub with a finger to prevent air embolization.
4. With the 16-gauge catheter in position, advance a 0.89 mm x 45 cm spring guide wire through the catheter. The guide wire should advance easily without resistance.
5. With the guide wire in position, remove the catheter, and use a No. 11 scalpel blade to nick the skin.
6. Place the central line catheter over the wire, holding the wire secure at all times. Pass the catheter into the vein, and suture the catheter with 2-0 silk suture, tape, and connect to an IV infusion.
7. Obtain a CXR to confirm position and rule out pneumothorax.

VI. Pulmonary Artery Catheterization Procedure

A. Using sterile technique, cannulate a vein using the technique above. The subclavian vein or internal jugular vein is commonly used.
B. Advance a guide wire through the cannula, then remove the cannula, but leave the guide wire in place. Keep the guide wire under control at all times. Nick the skin with a number 11-scalpel blade adjacent to the guide wire, and pass a number 8 French introducer over the wire into the vein. Remove the wire and connect the introducer to an IV fluid infusion, and suture with 2-0 silk.
C. Pass the proximal end of the pulmonary artery catheter (Swan Ganz) to an assistant for connection to a continuous flush transducer system.
D. Flush the distal and proximal ports with heparin solution, remove all bubbles, and check balloon integrity by inflating 2 cc of air. Check the pressure transducer by quickly moving the distal tip and watching monitor for response.
E. Pass the catheter through the introducer into the vein, then inflate the balloon with 1.0 cc of air, and advance the catheter until the balloon is in or near the right atrium.
F. The approximate distance to the entrance of the right atrium is determined from the site of insertion:
Right internal jugular vein: 10-15 cm.
Subclavian vein: 10 cm.
Femoral vein: 35.45 cm.
G. Advance the inflated balloon, while monitoring pressures and wave forms as the PA catheter is advanced. Watch for ventricular ectopy during insertion. Advance the catheter through the right ventricle into the main pulmonary artery until the catheter enters a distal branch of the pulmonary artery and is stopped (as evidenced by a pulmonary wedge pressure waveform).
H. Do not advance catheter while the balloon is deflated, and do not withdraw the catheter with the balloon inflated. After placement, obtain a chest X-ray to ensure that the tip of catheter is no farther than 3-5 cm from the mid-line, and no pneumothorax is present.

Normal Pulmonary Artery Catheter Values

Right atrial pressure	1-7 mmHg
RVP systolic	15-25 mmHg
RVP diastolic	8-15 mmHg
Pulmonary artery pressure	
PAP systolic	15-25 mmHg
PAP diastolic	8-15 mmHg
PAP mean	10-20 mmHg

16 Pulmonary Artery Catheter Values

Cardiovascular Disorders

John Roper, MD
Steve Marks, DO
Naeem Rana, MD

Myocardial Infarction

Each year 1.5 million people are diagnosed with an acute myocardial infarction.

I. Clinical evaluation of acute myocardial infarction
   A. Accurate diagnosis of acute myocardial infarction is based on clinical symptoms, electrocardiographic abnormalities and changes in the levels of serum markers of cardiac injury.
   B. Symptoms of MI may be characterized by a constricting or squeezing sensation in the chest. Pain can radiate to the upper abdomen, back, either arm, either shoulder, neck, or jaw.
   C. Nausea, vomiting, shortness of breath, diaphoresis, weakness, dizziness, palpitations, anxiety, or a sense of impending doom are also common.
   D. The presence of risk factors for coronary heart disease (age >45 in males, >55 in females, family history of coronary heart disease, smoking, hypertension, low HDL-cholesterol, diabetes), or a history of myocardial infarction should be assessed. Cardiac exam may reveal a third or fourth heart sound.

II. Differential diagnosis of chest pain
   A. **Acute pericarditis** is characterized by pleuritic-type chest pain and diffuse ST segment elevation on ECG.
   B. **Aortic dissection** is characterized by a "tearing" chest pain with uncontrolled hypertension, and widened mediastinum and increased aortic prominence on chest x-ray.
   C. **Esophageal rupture** usually occurs after forceful vomiting; x-ray may reveal air in mediastinum or a left side hydrothorax.
   D. **Acute peptic ulcer disease** manifests as epigastric pain with melena, or hematemesis and anemia.

III. Electrocardiographic findings in acute myocardial infarction
   A. ST-segment elevation in two adjacent leads is diagnostic of MI. The sensitivity and specificity are 49% and 92%, respectively.
   B. ST-segment depression is a nonspecific finding.
   C. Forty to 60 percent of patients who ultimately prove to have acute myocardial infarction have nondiagnostic ECGs.

IV. Laboratory testing
   A. Creatine kinase isoenzymes and CK isoforms
      1. Increased creatinine kinase, especially the isoenzyme CK-MB, is a sensitive sign of myocardial damage. Pathologic levels occur after 4 to 8 hours, and the peak occurs at 12 to 18 hours. Within the first four hours, the sensitivity of CK-MB for myocardial infarction is 25%.
      2. CK-MB produced in tissue is converted in plasma to $CK-MB^1$. At two to four hours after symptom onset, the presence of a $MB^2:MB^1$ ratio >1.5 has a sensitivity of 59%; at 4 to 6 hours, the sensitivity for myocardial infarction is 92%.

B. Troponins
1. Troponins are structural proteins that regulate actin and myosin in striated muscle. The main troponins are the cardiac isoforms of troponin T (c-TnT) and troponin I (c-TnI). Levels rise 3 to 12 hours after cardiac injury, and the levels remain elevated for 5 to 14 days. A rapid assay is available for c-TnT.
2. C-TnT is more specific for myocardial tissue than CK-MB (89% versus 63%); however, c-TnT also rises in patients with angina and may also rise in patients with muscular injury.

C. Myoglobin
1. Myoglobin is a protein found in both cardiac and skeletal muscle. It is detectable 1 to 4 hours after coronary occlusion, peaking at 6 to 9 hours and returning to baseline within 18 to 24 hours.
2. It is positive earlier than CK-MB, with a sensitivity at two hours of 23%, rising to 82% at two to four hours, and to 92% after four hours.

D. Lactic dehydrogenase is elevated at 25-48 hours, and it may be useful in patients who present late after onset of symptoms.

Serum Markers of Cardiac Injury				
Marker	Normal value	Rise after AMI	Peak Values	Return to Normal
Creatine kinase	<130 IU per L	4 to 8 hours	12 to 24 hours	4 to 5 days
CK-MB fraction	<13 IU per L	3 to 12 hours	10 to 18 hours	2 to 3 days
Lactic de-hydro-genase	<250 IU per L	24 to 48 hours	3 to 6 days	7 to 14 days
Myoglobin	<55 ng per mL	1 to 4 hours	6 to 9 hours	18 to 24 hours
C-TnT	Undetect-able	3 to 12 hours	12 to 24 hours and 2 to 3 days	5 to 14 days
C-TnI	Undetect-able	3 to 12 hours	24 hours	5 to 10 days

E. A fasting lipid profile should be obtained. Lipid measurements are valid for up to 8 hours after admission for MI.

V. **Emergent therapy for myocardial infarction**
   A. **Primary percutaneous transluminal angioplasty** is the most efficient method of restoring blood flow and conserving heart muscle. Primary angioplasty in patients with anterior MI results in a higher survival rate, lower rates of stroke, reinfarction and recurrent ischemia than does thrombolysis. The American College of Cardiology recommends primary PTCA in the following situations:
   1. If performed within a few hours of symptom onset.

  2. In patients with cardiogenic shock.
  3. In patients at risk of bleeding or other contraindications for thrombolytic therapy.

B. Indications for thrombolytic therapy in myocardial infarction
  1. All patients who have had more than 20 minutes or angina refractory to sublingual nitroglycerin, associated with ≥ 0.1 mV of ST-segment elevation, in two or more contiguous leads, should be considered for thrombolytic therapy.
  2. Patients with a new left bundle branch block and a history suggesting acute myocardial infarction should also receive thrombolytic therapy.

C. Contraindications
  1. Active internal bleeding (not including menses).
  2. History of cerebrovascular hemorrhage or emboli.
  3. Recent intracranial or intraspinal surgery or trauma.
  4. Intracranial neoplasm, arteriovenous malformation, or aneurysm.
  5. Known bleeding diathesis.
  6. Severe uncontrolled hypertension ≥ 180 mmHg ststolic and/or ≥ 110 mmHg diastolic.

D. Relative contraindications
  1. History of prior cerebrovascular accident or known intracerebral disease not covered in contraindications.
  2. Current use of anticoagulants in therapeutic doses (INR ≥ 2.0-3.0); known bleeding diathesis
  3. Recent (within 2-4 weeks) trauma, including head injury, traumatic or prolonged (>10 min) CPR, or major surgery (<3 wk).
  4. Non-compressible vascular punctures.
  5. Recent (within 2-4 weeks) internal bleeding.
  6. For use of streptokinase: prior exposure (within 5 days to 1 yr) or prior allergic reaction.
  7. Pregnancy
  8. Active peptic ulcer disease
  9. History of chronic severe hypertension.

E. Streptokinase (Streptase)
  1. Streptokinase is the least expensive thrombolytic; it offers about the same benefit as tPA, except in those who present with an anterior MI within 4 hours of chest pain.
  2. Streptokinase IV infusion: 1.5 million IU in 100 mL NS IV over 60 min. Administer methylprednisolone (Solu-Medrol), 250 mg IVP, and diphenhydramine (Benadryl), 50 mg IVP, prior to streptokinase.

F. Reteplase (Retavase) 10 U IV push over 2 min. Repeat second 10 U IV push in 30 minutes. The 90 min patency rate is greater with reteplase than with alteplase; however, the 30-day mortality is the same.

G. Alteplase (tissue plasminogen activator, tPA, Activase)
  1. The 90 min patency rate is greater with tPA than SK, but there is no difference at 24 hours.
  2. IV bolus of 15 mg, then 0.75 mg/kg (up to 50 mg) over 30 min, followed by 0.5 mg/kg (up to 35 mg) infused over the next 60 min.

VI. Drug therapy for acute myocardial infarction
A. Aspirin
  1. Patients with any sign of an acute coronary syndrome should immediately chew and swallow 325 mg of aspirin, followed by 160

mg PO qd on subsequent days. During recovery, the dosage can be decreased to 80 mg per day.

2. Aspirin decreases the relative risk of mortality by 25% after MI.

B. Heparin

1. Heparin has no influence on mortality; however, it reduces the frequency of ischemic events and reocclusion after thrombolysis. Heparin should be continued for at least 48 hours.

2. Use of heparin after reteplase and alteplase (tPA) is mandatory; however, heparin is optional after streptokinase. All patients at risk for systemic emboli (previous embolus, atrial fibrillation, left ventricular thrombus, large anterior MI) should receive heparin.

3. Heparin 5000 U IVP is given before thrombolysis. The initial bolus of heparin is followed by heparin 10 units/kg/h if alteplase (tPA) or streptokinase was given. The initial bolus of heparin is followed by heparin 15 units/kg/h if reteplase was given. Titrate heparin to aPTT of 50-70 seconds.

C. Nitrates

1. Intravenous nitroglycerin should be given to patients with suspected MI or unstable angina unless hypotension is present.

2. Initial administration consists of a 12.5-25 mcg bolus, followed by 10-20 mcg/min, titrated to chest pain. The dose can be increased as needed to 200 mcg/min.

3. Nitroglycerin should be continue for 24-48 hours. Thereafter, if the patient is free of chest pain, it should be tapered and discontinued. Oral or transdermal nitrates should be substituted for IV nitroglycerin after stabilization. Sublingual nitroglycerin may also be given initially (0.4 mg SL q5min prn chest pain).

4. **Contraindications** to nitroglycerin include a systolic blood pressure <90 mm Hg and a heart rate <50 beats per minute.

D. Beta-blockers

1. Patients should receive a beta-blocker within 12 hours of onset of myocardial infarction and continued for 3 months, unless contraindicated.

2. **Contraindications** include bradycardia, second- or third-degree atrioventricular block, hypotension, evidence of congestive heart failure (rales, audible S_3), cardiogenic shock, and active bronchospasm.

3. **Atenolol (Tenormin)**, 5 mg IV, repeated in 5 minutes, followed by 50-100 mg PO qd.

4. **Metoprolol (Lopressor)**, 5 mg IV push every 5 minutes for three doses; followed by 25 mg PO bid. Titrate up to 100 mg PO bid.

E. Morphine sulfate. Analgesia with morphine (2-4 mg IVP prn chest pain) should also be provided.

F. Angiotensin converting enzyme inhibitors

1. ACE-inhibitors improve survival and decrease morbidity in patients with left ventricular dysfunction (ejection fraction <40%) after myocardial infarction.

2. An oral angiotensin-converting-enzyme (ACE) inhibitor should be initiated within 24 hours after the onset of myocardial infarction in patients with a large anterior myocardial infarction or with evidence of left ventricular dysfunction. An echocardiogram should be used to

evaluate left ventricular function before discharge in all patients with a transmural Q wave infarction.

3. Captopril (Capoten) is given as an initial dose of 6.25 mg PO, and 4-6 hours later the dosage should be increased to 12.5 mg q8h. Gradually increase to 25-50 mg PO q8h.

4. Enalapril (Vasotec) 2.5 mg PO qd; titrate to 10-20 mg PO qd.

5. ACE-inhibitor therapy should not begin until the patient's condition has stabilized.

6. **Contraindications to ACE-inhibitors:** Systolic blood pressure under 100 mm Hg, clinical renal failure, significant valvular stenosis, bilateral stenosis of the renal arteries, known allergy to the drugs.

7. ACE-inhibitor treatment may be stopped at 4-6 weeks in patients with normal left ventricular systolic function. It should be continued indefinitely in patients with a low ejection fraction (<40%).

G. **Calcium channel blockers** have no role in the routine management of acute MI except in situations where beta blockers are ineffective or contraindicated, such as in patients with bronchospasm.

H. **Magnesium** has not been shown to produce a benefit in MI, and it should not be used routinely for MI, except to correct hypomagnesemia.
§

Congestive Heart Failure

Heart failure is a develops when cardiac output becomes insufficient to meet systemic metabolic demands. Left ventricular systolic dysfunction can be recognized by the presence of a left ventricular ejection fraction less than 40%.

I. **Clinical evaluation of heart failure**

A. **Symptoms** of heart failure include paroxysmal nocturnal dyspnea, orthopnea, and new-onset dyspnea on exertion.

B. **Chest pain** may indicate that ischemia is the cause of heart failure; however, ischemia can also occur without chest pain.

C. **Past history** of a heart murmur, prior viral illness, hypertension, myocardial infarction, alcohol or drug use, thyroid disease, or lung disease should be sought.

D. **Precipitating cause.** The most common precipitating cause of CHF is lack of compliance with dietary and medical regimens. Atrial fibrillation sometimes exacerbates CHF. Nonsteroidal anti-inflammatory agents, alcohol, hyperthyroidism, and beta blockers (including eyedrops) can exacerbate CHF.

E. **Assessment of functional capacity** reflects on the effectiveness of therapy. Capacity to perform activities, such as climbing one or two flights of stairs or walking 50 or 100 feet should be assessed.

II. **Physical examination**

A. **Vital signs, mental status, capillary refill, urine output, and skin temperature** should be assessed.

B. **Auscultation of the lungs and evaluation of jugular vein distention** allows rapid assessment of volume status and filling pressures.

C. **Right ventricular failure**, which often accompanies right ventricular infarction, usually causes systemic hypotension, increased jugular vein distention, and signs of hypoperfusion.

D. **Left ventricular failure** almost always causes pulmonary crackles.

E. **Palpation of ventricular impulses and auscultation of heart sounds** can uncover acute valvular insufficiency (regurgitant murmur), hypertensive heart disease (sustained left ventricular impulse and S4), and chronic left ventricular dysfunction (diffuse and dyskinetic left ventricular impulse with an S3).

Conditions That Mimic or Provoke Heart Failure

Coronary artery disease and myocardial infarction	Tachyarrhythmias or bradyarrhythmias
Hypertension	Pulmonary embolism
Aortic or mitral valve disease	Pulmonary disease
Cardiomyopathies: Hypertrophic, idiopathic dilated, postpartum, genetic, toxic, nutritional, metabolic	Congenital abnormalities
	High output states: Anemia, hyperthyroidism
Myocarditis: Infectious, toxic, immune	A-V fistulas, Paget's disease, fibrous dysplasia, multiple myeloma
Pericardial constriction	Renal failure, nephrotic syndrome

Laboratory Evaluation of Heart Failure

Echocardiogram, CXR, EKG
Electrolytes, BUN, creatinine, calcium, albumin
CBC, urinalysis
Thyroid stimulating hormone should be assessed if there is atrial fibrillation, evidence of thyroid disease, or age >65 yrs.

Clinical Evaluation of Laboratory Studies

Test	Finding	Possible Diagnosis
Electrocardiogram	Acute ST-T wave changes	Myocardial ischemia
	Atrial fibrillation, other tachyarrhythmia	Thyroid disease or heart failure due to rapid ventricular rate
	Bradyarrhythmias	Heart failure due to low heart rate
	Previous myocardial infarction (Q waves)	Heart failure due to reduced left ventricular performance.
	Low voltage	Pericardial effusion
	Left ventricular hypertrophy	Diastolic dysfunction
Complete blood count	Anemia	Heart failure due decreased oxygen-carrying capacity
Urinalysis	Proteinuria	Nephrotic syndrome
Serum creatinine	Elevated	Renal failure
Thyroid-stimulating hormone	Abnormal	Heart failure due to hypothyroidism or hyperthyroidism

F. **Chest roentgenogram.** The chest film can help differentiate patients with a normal-sized heart and pulmonary edema, suggesting newly developing acute heart failure secondary to acute myocardial infarction or valvular insufficiency, from patients with an enlarged cardiac silhouette, suggesting an acute exacerbation of chronic CHF.

G. **Electrocardiography** may identify acute myocardial infarction and often dictates whether the patient is a candidate for thrombolytic therapy. It may reveal evidence of an old myocardial infarction, hypertrophy, and/or conduction system delays.

H. **Echocardiography**

1. Echocardiography is used to differentiate between left ventricular systolic dysfunction, left ventricular diastolic dysfunction, valvular heart disease, or a non-cardiac etiology.

2. Most patients with heart failure are found to have ejection fractions of less than 40%.

I. **Assessment of ischemia**

1. **Ischemic heart disease** is a potentially reversible cause of heart failure. Risk factors for coronary disease, history of prior infarction and history of angina should be sought. Non-invasive stress testing, using exercise or dobutamine stress electrocardiography, should assess regional wall motion abnormalities in patients with unexplained heart failure.

2. If non-invasive testing suggests underlying coronary artery disease, the evaluation should proceed to coronary arteriography.

III. **Management of congestive heart failure**

A. **Angiotensin converting enzyme inhibitors and angiotensin-II receptor blockers**

1. For patients with left ventricular systolic dysfunction without overt clinical volume overload, ACE-inhibitors should be prescribed unless contraindicated (potassium level >5.5 mmol/L, symptomatic hypotension). Diuretics should be added if symptoms persist despite maximal treatment with ACE inhibitors.

2. If there is overt clinical volume overload (pulmonary edema, ankle edema or exertional dyspnea), both an ACE inhibitor and a diuretic should be added simultaneously.

3. The ACE-inhibitor should be given at a maximum tolerable dose. A systolic BP of 90 mmHg is acceptable unless significant coronary artery disease is present.

4. **Side effects of ACE-inhibitors** include postural hypotension, renal insufficiency, and hyperkalemia. Development of a chronic dry cough is common.

5. Angiotensin-II receptor blockers may be used in place of an ACE-inhibitor if cough, angioedema, or rash develops.

Drug Treatment of Heart Failure

Drug	Initial Dose	Target Dose	Max Dose	Adverse Reactions
ACE Inhibitors				
Enalapril (Vasotec)	2.5 mg bid	10 mg bid	20 mg bid	Hypotension, hyperkalemia, renal insufficiency, cough, skin rash, angioedema, neutropenia
Lisinopril (Prinivil, Zestril)	5 mg qd	20 mg qd	40 mg qd	Same as enalapril
Quinapril (Accupril)	5 mg bid	20 mg bid	20 mg bid	Same as enalapril
Ramipril (Altace)	2.5 bid	5 mg bid	10 mg bid	Same as enalapril
Angiotensin-II Receptor Blockers				
Irbesartan (Avapro)	75 mg qd	150 mg qd	300 mg qd	Hypotension
Losartan (Cozaar)	25 mg bid	50 mg bid	50 mg bid	Hyperkalemia in azotemia
Valsartan (Diovan)	80 mg qd	80 mg bid	160 mg bid	Hypotension
Beta-Blockers				
Carvedilol (Coreg)	3.125 mg bid	12.5 mg bid	25 mg bid	Lower extremity edema
Metoprolol (Lopressor)	6.25 mg bid	50 mg bid	100 mg bid	Rash, pruritus
Bisoprolol (Zebeta)	2.5 mg qd	10 mg qd	20 mg qd	Fatigue
Digitalis Glycoside				
Digoxin (Lanoxin)	0.125 mg qd	0.125-0.5 mg qd	0.5 mg qd	Atrioventricular block, ventricular tachycardia or fibrillation, nausea, yellow-green halos

Drug	Initial Dose	Target Dose	Max Dose	Adverse Reactions
Loop Diuretics				
Furosemide (Lasix)	10-40 mg qd	40-80 mg qd-bid	240 mg bid	Postural hypotension, hypokalemia, hyperglycemia, hyperuricemia, rash; rarely pancreatitis, bone marrow suppression
Torsemide (Demadex)	5-10 mg qd	20-40 mg qd	100 mg bid	Same as furosemide
Bumetanide (Bumex)	0.5 mg qd	1-2 mg qd	2 mg bid	Same as furosemide
Nitrates				
Nitroglycerin IV	10 mcg/min	Advance to 5-130 mcg/min in 5-10 mcg/min increments.		Headache and hypotension
Nitroprusside	0.1-5.0 mcg/kg/min IV			Thiocyanate or cyanide toxicity at high doses in azotemia
Isosorbide dinitrate (Isordil)	10 mg tid	20 mg tid	40 mg tid	Headache, hypotension
Isosorbide mononitrate (ISMO, Imdur)	20 mg qd 30 mg qd	20 mg bid 60 mg qd	20 mg bid 120 mg qd	Headache, dizziness, hypotension
Vasodilators				
Hydralazine (Apresoline)	25 mg tid-qid	50 mg qid	100 mg tid	Lupus-like syndrome, tachycardia

B. Inotropic therapy–digoxin

1. Digoxin increases ventricular contractility in patients with left ventricular systolic dysfunction.
2. Patients with mild to moderate heart failure will often become asymptomatic with ACE inhibitors, and these patients do not require digoxin. Digoxin should be added to the regimen if symptoms persist despite optimal doses of ACE inhibitors.
3. In patients with severe heart failure, digoxin should be initiated along with ACE inhibitors and diuretics.

     4. Digoxin is ineffective and contraindicated in patients who have preserved systolic function, reduced ventricular compliance, and diastolic dysfunction.

C. Diuretics

    1. Diuretics are useful for reducing symptoms of volume overload (orthopnea, paroxysmal nocturnal dyspnea). Diuretics should be started immediately when patients present with symptoms or signs of volume overload. Diuretics reduce intravascular volume and preload.

    2. Loop diuretics (furosemide, torsemide) are diuretics of first choice. Severe congestive symptoms may require a twice daily regimen because of fluid accumulation during the day. Torsemide has greater oral absorption and a longer duration of action than furosemide.

    3. Adverse effects. Orthostatic hypotension or abnormalities of fluid and electrolyte balance (hypokalemia, hypomagnesemia) occur. Serum magnesium and potassium levels should be monitored and supplemented when necessary.

D. Nitrates. Nitrates improve the symptoms of pulmonary congestion by reducing preload.

E. Beta-blockers

    1. Long-term use of beta-adrenergic blockers improves survival and significantly improves ejection fraction in patients with mild to moderate heart failure.

    2. Carvedilol (Coreg)

        a. This beta-blocker improves long-term survival by 65% in heart failure patients. It is approved for treatment of mild to moderate failure.

        b. Carvedilol should be initiated at a low dosage of 3.125 mg bid, and increased slowly to 6.25-50 mg bid.

    3. Metoprolol (Lopressor) 6.25 mg PO bid. Titrate to 50-100 mg bid.

    4. Bisoprolol (Zebeta) 2.5 mg PO qd. Titrate to 10-20 mg qd.

F. Inotropic agents for persistent hypotension and cardiogenic shock

    1. Cardiogenic shock has a mortality rate of 85%. In patients who are progressing toward shock, dobutamine at 5-15 mcg/kg/min or dopamine at 2-5 mcg/kg/min may improve clinical status.

    2. Milrinone (Primacor). Initial dose is 50 mcg/kg IV over 10 min, then 0.375 mg/kg/min with titration to 0.75 mcg/kg/min. Milrinone may cause hypotension, atrial fibrillation or ventricular arrhythmias.

    3. In patients who are severely hypotensive ($\leq$70 mmHg) with volume overload, moderate (4-5 mcg/kg/min) doses of dopamine may improve cardiac output without causing systemic vasoconstriction.

    4. Intra-aortic balloon counterpulsation should be considered to support circulation.

IV. Non-pharmacologic measures

    A. Patients should be able to recognize the symptoms of worsening heart failure, and they should check their weight daily. If a worsening of symptoms or a weight gain of 3-5 lb or more within one week occurs, the patient should take an extra dose of diuretic.

    B. Regular exercise should be encouraged.

    C. Dietary therapy. Dietary sodium should be restricted to 3 g per day. Fluid restriction is not advisable unless hyponatremia is present. Alcohol should be limited to no more than one drink per day. §

Atrial Fibrillation

Atrial fibrillation is the most frequently encountered cardiac arrhythmia, with a prevalence of 2%. In patients older than 65 years old, the prevalence is 5%.

I. **Clinical evaluation**

   A. Atrial fibrillation (AF) may manifest only as fatigue caused by impaired cardiac output or the patient may have no symptoms. Palpitations, shortness of breath or chest pain may occur, and syncope may infrequently accompany AF. Symptoms of myocardial ischemia and angina may be caused by the rapid ventricular rate. Paroxysmal AF may cause symptoms that abate and recur.

   B. The cause of the atrial fibrillation should be identified. Precipitating causes, such as hyperthyroidism, electrolyte abnormalities, and drug toxicity, should be excluded. Stimulant abuse, excess tobacco, alcohol, caffeine, chocolate, over-the-counter cold remedies, and street drugs should be sought. AF may be associated with a recent acute illness, such as pneumonia.

II. **Physical examination**

   A. The pulse is characterized by an irregular-irregular timing and amplitude. The rapid ventricular rate may cause hypotension and pulmonary congestion.

   B. The patient should be examined for hypertension, rheumatic fever, valvular disease, pericarditis, coronary artery disease, hyperthyroidism, or chronic obstructive pulmonary disease.

   C. Murmurs and cardiac enlargement should be sought. Peripheral bruits may be a marker for associated coronary artery disease.

III. **Diagnostic evaluation**

   A. **12-lead electrocardiogram** reveals irregular R-R intervals with no P waves. The ventricular rate is irregularly, irregular and the ventricular response rate is usually 130-180 bpm.

   B. **Laboratory evaluation.** Chest x-ray, electrolytes and screening labs, ECG, transesophageal echocardiogram, free T4, TSH, and drug levels (theophylline) should be assessed.

Causes of Atrial Fibrillation	
Hypoglycemia	Hypertrophic cardiomyopathy
Theophylline intoxication	Coronary artery disease
Acute pulmonary disease (pneumonia, asthma, chronic obstructive pulmonary disease, pulmonary embolus)	Atrial septal defect
	Aortic stenosis
	Infiltrative diseases (amyloidosis, cardiac tumors)
Heavy alcohol intake or alcohol withdrawal	Acute myocardial infarction
Hyperthyroidism	Lone atrial fibrillation (No underlying disease state)
Severe acute systemic illness	Electrolyte abnormalities
Left or right ventricular failure	Stimulant abuse, excess tobacco, xanthine (tea), chocolate, over-the-counter cold remedies, street drugs.
Mitral valve disease (stenosis or regurgitation)	
Pericarditis	
Hypertensive heart disease with left ventricular hypertrophy	

IV. Emergency management of unstable atrial fibrillation

A. Treatment of patients with acute hypotension, angina or heart failure

1. Immediate direct-current cardioversion should be administered in unstable patients. Anesthesia or sedation and supplemental oxygen should be initiated if time permits.
2. After cardioversion, rhythm should be stabilized with an oral antiarrhythmic.

V. Initial management of the patient with stable atrial fibrillation

A. Acute rate control

1. Immediate control of the ventricular rate is the first goal in patients who do not require immediate cardioversion. Ventricular rate should usually be brought to below 100/min.

2. **Calcium channel blockers**
   a. Diltiazem (Cardizem) is the a preferred rate control agent because of rapid onset of action. Dosage is 0.25 mg/kg (20 mg) IV bolus over 2 min, followed by an infusion of 5-15 mg/h, titrated to heart rate. The bolus may be repeated with 0.35 mg/kg if needed.
   b. Verapamil (Calan) 2.5-5 mg IVP q4-6h is also effective.
   c. Calcium blockers are contraindicated in CHF or high grade atrioventricular block.

3. **Beta blockers**
   a. Beta-blockers are also used for acute rate control. Contraindications include asthma, obstructive lung disease, and heart failure.
   b. **Propranolol (Inderal)**: 1-4 mg IV at 1 mg/min. A second dose may be given after 2 minutes if necessary. Maintenance: 10-30 mg PO tid-qid.
   c. **Metoprolol (Lopressor)** 5 mg IV doses; 25-100 mg PO bid.

4. **Digoxin** is appropriate only in patients with left ventricular systolic dysfunction. Six hours are required before rate control can be accomplished. Digoxin does not promote conversion to normal sinus rhythm. Loading dose: 0.5 mg IV/PO, then 0.25 mg IV q4h x 2-3 doses, followed by 0.125-0.25 mg/day IV/PO.

VI. Intermediate management of stable atrial fibrillation

A. Restoration of sinus rhythm

1. After the ventricular rate has been controlled, restoration of sinus rhythm should be accomplished because rate control improves cardiac output and reduces the risk of systemic embolization.
2. Sinus rhythm can be restored by IV loading of an antiarrhythmic drug (procainamide or ibutilide) or an oral agent, such as quinidine or disopyramide. If pharmacologic conversion is ineffective, elective, direct-current cardioversion should be initiated.

B. Anticoagulation

1. If transesophageal echocardiography (TEE) has excluded the presence of an atrial thrombus, the patient may be cardioverted to sinus rhythm without anticoagulation.
2. If TEE reveals an atrial thrombus, warfarin (Coumadin) should be administered for 3 weeks before the cardioversion, to an INR of 2.0-3.0. After successful cardioversion, warfarin is continued for 4 weeks.

VII. Elective direct-current cardioversion
   A. The ventricular rate should be controlled and the patient anticoagulated before elective cardioversion if AF has been present for more than 48 hours.
   B. Conversion usually is accomplished with 200 to 300 Joules, but up to 360 J may be required.

VIII. Antiarrhythmic drug therapy
   A. Antiarrythmic agents (class Ia, Ic, III) are all effective in achieving a sinus rhythm to varying degrees. They have not been shown to reduce stroke risk or to reduce overall mortality and have been associated with a small risk for life-threatening proarrythmia.
   B. Class Ia antiarrhythmic drugs
   1. Procainamide (Pronestyl)
      a. It is a preferred agent for acute pharmacologic cardioversion unless an autoimmune disorder is present. The conversion rate is 43-58%.
      b. Loading dose is 15 mg/kg (1000 mg) IV over 20 minutes, followed by an infusion of 2-4 mg/min (2 gm in 250 mL D5W = 8 mg/mL). The patient should be monitored for hypotension, QRS widening, and QT prolongation.
      c. Long-term therapy with procainamide may cause arthritis, rash, or a lupus-like syndrome.
   2. Quinidine gluconate (Quinaglute). Conversion rate is 50-60%. Forty to 50% of patients can not tolerate quinidine because of diarrhea. The dosage is 324 mg PO tid-qid.
   3. Disopyramide (Norpace) has potent negative inotropic and anticholinergic properties. It is not recommended in older men because of urinary retention. 100-300 mg of the SR cap PO bid.
   C. Class Ic antiarrhythmic drugs
   1. Flecainide and propafenone are associated with excess mortality in patients post MI, and they have significant proarrhythmic properties in patients with LV dysfunction.
   2. Flecainide is highly effective for controlling atrial fibrillation with structurally normal hearts; 50-100 mg PO q12h; max 200 mg q12h. It should be avoided in patients with ischemia or LV dysfunction.
   3. Propafenone: 150-225 mg PO q8h; max 400 mg PO q8h.
   D. Class III antiarrhythmics
   1. Amiodarone (Cordarone)
      a. Amiodarone is more effective and better tolerated than class Ia agents, particularly in the presence of left ventricular dysfunction. Loading dose is 400 mg bid PO for 2 weeks; then reduce to 400 mg qd for one month, then reduce to maintenance of 200 qd.
      b. Amiodarone is the most effective antiarrhythmic at maintaining sinus rhythm. It is 78% effective at maintaining sinus rhythm in people who had failed a type-I antiarrhythmic.
      c. Toxicities include hepatic dysfunction, pneumonitis, hyperthyroidism, hypothyroidism, and skin hyperpigmentation. Reversible pulmonary toxicity develops in 10-17% of patients receiving more than 400 mg/day.
   2. Ibutilide (Corvert). The conversion rate is 30-40%. It is used for acute pharmacologic conversion; 1 mg IV over 10 min; may repeat

dose after 10-15 minutes. Torsades de pointes arrhythmia occurs in 8% of patients.

3. Sotalol (Betapace)
a. Sotalol has significant beta-blocking activity, and it may cause bradycardia and Torsades de pointes arrhythmia. Sotalol is as effective as quinidine, and it offers both rate control and antiarrhythmic properties. It is contraindicated in CHF and asthma.

b. Initial dosage: 80 mg PO bid, increasing prn to 240-320 mg/d, divided bid-tid.

E. Maintenance antiarrhythmic therapy

1. **Patients with no structural heart disease**. If the patient does not have structural heart disease, flecainide is recommended. Sotalol is also effective, and amiodarone can be used if other agents fail.

2. **Ischemic heart disease**
a. Sotalol is recommended because it has beta-blocking properties. Amiodarone can be used if other agents fail.

b. The class 1C drugs (flecainide, propafenone) should be avoided because of increased mortality in patients with ischemia.

3. **Congestive heart failure or left ventricular dysfunction**
a. Amiodarone is the best drug in these patients because it has the least negative inotropic effect.

b. In the patients with CHF and LV dysfunction, class 1C agents should be used with caution because of proarrhythmic properties.

c. Nonpharmacologic approaches should be considered because increased LV function often results from rate control.

IX. Non-pharmacological approaches to atrial fibrillation

A. **Catheter ablation and ventricular pacing** is a highly effective modality in patients who have failed pharmacologic approaches.

B. **Surgical treatment of atrial fibrillation.** The Maze procedure consists of multiple atriotomies which interrupt the re-entrant circuits.

X. Stroke prevention therapy for patients with chronic atrial fibrillation

A. Patients with chronic atrial fibrillation have a 6-fold increased risk of stroke. Warfarin reduces the risk of stroke. Aspirin is less effective than warfarin for preventing stroke.

B. **Risk factors for stroke** include age >65 years, previous stroke or transient ischemic attack, hypertension, diabetes, heart failure, myocardial ischemia, or valvular disease.

C. **Indications for antithrombotic therapy in chronic atrial fibrillation**
1. **Patients with a strong contraindication to warfarin** should receive aspirin 325 mg per day.

2. **Patients less than 65 with lone atrial fibrillation** should receive no treatment or they should receive aspirin.

3. **Patients with no risk factors for stroke** should receive aspirin.

4. **Patients with one or more risk factors for stroke** should be treated with warfarin, titrated to an INR of 2.0-3.0.

5. **Patients 70 years of age or older and low-risk** should receive warfarin, titrated to an INR of 2.0, or they should receive aspirin. §

Hypertensive Emergency

Hypertensive crises are characterized by severe elevations in blood pressure (BP). Then diastolic blood pressure (BP) is usually higher than 120 mmHg to 130 mmHg.

I. **Clinical Evaluation of Hypertensive Crises**

    A. **Hypertensive emergency** is defined by a diastolic blood pressure >120 mmHg associated with ongoing vascular damage. Symptoms or signs of neurologic, cardiac, renal, or retinal dysfunction are present. Hypertensive emergencies include severe hypertension in the following settings:

        1. Aortic dissection

        2. Acute left ventricular failure and pulmonary edema

        3. Acute renal failure or worsening of chronic renal failure

        4. Hypertensive encephalopathy

        5. Focal neurologic damage indicating thrombotic or hemorrhagic stroke

        6. Pheochromocytoma, cocaine overdose, or other hyperadrenergic states

        7. Unstable angina or myocardial infarction

        8. Eclampsia

    B. **Hypertensive urgency** is defined as diastolic blood pressure >120 mmHg without evidence of vascular damage; the disorder is asymptomatic and no retinal lesions are present.

    C. **Causes of secondary hypertension** include renovascular hypertension, pheochromocytoma, cocaine use, withdrawal from alpha$_2$ stimulants, clonidine, beta blockers or alcohol, and noncompliance with antihypertensive medications.

II. **Initial Assessment of Severe Hypertension**

    A. When severe hypertension is noted, the measurement should be repeated in both arms to detect any significant differences.

    B. Peripheral pulses should be assessed for absence or delay, which suggests a dissecting aortic dissection. Evidence of pulmonary edema should be sought.

    C. Target organ damage is suggested by chest pain, neurologic signs, altered mental status, profound headache, dyspnea, abdominal pain, hematuria, focal neurologic signs (paralysis or paresthesia), or hypertensive retinopathy.

    D. Prescription drug use should be assessed, including missed doses of antihypertensives. History of recent cocaine or amphetamine use should be sought.

    E. If focal neurologic signs are present, a CT scan may be required to differentiate hypertensive encephalopathy from a stroke syndrome. In stroke syndromes, hypertension may be secondary to the neurologic event; the neurologic deficits are fixed and follow a predictable neuroanatomic pattern. By contrast, in hypertensive encephalopathy, the neurologic signs follow no anatomic pattern, and there is diffuse alteration in mental function.

III. **Laboratory Evaluation**

    A. Complete blood cell count, urinalysis for protein, glucose, and blood; urine sediment examination for cells, casts, and bacteria; chemistry panel (SMA-18).

    B. If chest pain is present, cardiac enzymes are obtained.

C. If the history suggests a hyperadrenergic state, the possibility of a pheochromocytoma should be excluded with a 24 hour urine catecholamines. A urine drug screen may be necessary to exclude illicit drug use.

D. Electrocardiogram.

E. Suspected primary aldosteronism can be excluded with a 24 hour urine potassium and an assessment of plasma renin activity. Renal artery stenosis can be excluded with captopril renography and intravenous pyelography.

Screening Tests for Secondary Hypertension	
Renovascular Hypertension	Captopril Test: Plasma renin level before and 1 hr after captopril 25 mg PO. A greater than 150% increase in renin is positive Captopril Renography: Renal scan before and after 25 mg PO Intravenous Pyelography MRI Angiography
Hyperaldosteronism	Serum Potassium 24 hr Urine Potassium Plasma Renin Activity CT Scan of Adrenals
Pheochromocytoma	24 hr Urine Catecholamines CT Scan Nuclear MIBG Scan
Cushing's Syndrome	Plasma ACTH Dexamethasone Suppression Test
Hyperparathyroidism	Serum Calcium Serum Parathyroid hormone

IV. Management of Hypertensive Emergencies

A. The patient should be hospitalized for bed rest, intravenous access, continuous intra-arterial blood pressure monitoring, and electrocardiographic monitoring. Volume status and urinary output should be monitored.

B. Rapid, uncontrolled reductions in blood pressure should be avoided because coma, stroke, myocardial infarction, acute renal failure, or death may result.

C. The goal of initial therapy is to terminate ongoing target organ damage. The MAP should be lowered not more than 20-25%, or to a diastolic blood pressure of 100 mmHg.

D. In hypertensive crises associated with myocardial ischemia, acute left ventricular failure or dissection of the aorta, treatment should be more aggressive and blood pressure lowered within 15 to 30 minutes.

V. Parenteral Antihypertensive Agents

A. Nitroprusside (Nipride)

1. Nitroprusside is the drug of choice in almost all hypertensive emergencies (except myocardial ischemia or renal impairment). It dilates both arteries and veins, and it reduces afterload and preload.

2. Onset of action is nearly instantaneous, and the effects disappear approximately 1-10 minutes after discontinuation.
3. The starting dosage is 0.25-1.0 mcg/kg/min by continuous infusion with a range of 0.25-8.0 mcg/kg/min. Titrate dose to gradually reduce blood pressure.
4. When treatment is prolonged or when renal insufficiency is present, the risk of cyanide and thiocyanate toxicity is increased. Signs of thiocyanate toxicity include anorexia, disorientation, fatigue, hallucinations, nausea, toxic psychosis, and seizures. Clinical deterioration with cyanosis, metabolic acidosis and arrhythmias indicates cyanide toxicity.

B. Nitroglycerin

1. Nitroglycerin is the drug of choice for hypertensive emergencies with coronary ischemia. It should not be used with hypertensive encephalopathy because it increases intracranial pressure.
2. Nitroglycerin increases venous capacitance, decreases venous return and left ventricular filling pressure. It has a rapid onset of action of 2-5 minutes. Tolerance may occur within 24-48 hours.
3. The starting dose is 15 mcg IV bolus, then 5-10 mcg/min (50 mg in 250 mL D5W). Titrate by increasing the dose at 3-5-minute intervals up to max 1.0 mcg/kg/min.

C. Labetalol IV (Normodyne)

1. Labetalol is a good choice if BP elevation is associated with hyperadrenergic activity, aortic dissection, or postoperative hypertension. It is also an excellent choice for patients with aortic or abdominal aneurysm.
2. It is administered as 20 mg slow IV over 2 min. Additional doses of 20-80 mg may be administered q5-10min, then q3-4h prn or 0.5-2.0 mg/min IV infusion.
3. The onset of action is 5 minutes, and maximum effect occurs 30 minutes after each dose. Effects persist for 3-6 hours.
4. Labetalol is contraindicated in obstructive pulmonary disease, decompensated CHF, or heart block greater than first degree.

D. Enalaprilat IV (Vasotec)

1. Enalaprilat is an ACE-inhibitor with a rapid onset of action (15 min) and long duration of action (11 hours). It is ideal for patients with heart failure or accelerated-malignant hypertension.
2. Initial dose 1.25 mg IVP (over 2-5 min) q6h, then increase up to 5 mg q6h. Adjust dose in azotemic patients. Do not use in presence of renal artery stenosis.

E. Nicardipine IV (Cardene IV)

1. Nicardipine is a fast-acting calcium channel blocker that shares many of the predictable antihypertensive qualities of nitroprusside.
2. Infusion is started at 5 mg/h and may be increased to 15 mg/h; BP is usually controlled at 7.5 mg/h. Its onset of action is 5-10 minutes and effects cease 10-15 minutes after discontinuation.

F. Phentolamine (Regitine) is an intravenous alpha-adrenergic antagonist used in excess catecholamine states, such as pheochromocytomas, rebound hypertension due to withdrawal of clonidine, and drug ingestions. The dose is 2-5 mg IV every 5 to 10 minutes.

G. Trimethaphan (Arfonad) is a ganglionic-blocking agent that blocks both adrenergic and cholinergic ganglia. It is useful in dissecting aortic

aneurysm when beta blockers are contraindicated; however, it is rarely used. The dose is 0.3-3 mg/min IV infusion. The onset of action is 1-5 minutes and tachyphylaxis occurs within 48 hours. §

Ventricular Arrhythmias

I. Ventricular fibrillation and tachycardia
  -**If unstable (see ACLS protocol page 5)**, defibrillate with unsynchronized 200 J, 300 J, then 360 J.
  -Oxygen 100% by mask.
  -Lidocaine loading dose 50-100 mg IV, then 2-4 mg/min IV **OR**
  -Bretylium loading dose 5-10 mg/kg over 5-10 min, then 2-4 mg/min IV (may repeat loading dose up to total 30 mg/kg.
  -Amiodarone 150 mg over 10min, then 1 mg/min x 6 hours, then 0.5 mg/min IV infusion.
  -Procainamide loading dose 10-15 mg/kg at 20 mg/min IV or 100 mg IV q5min, then 2-4 mg/min IV maintenance **OR**
  -**Also see "other antiarrhythmics" below.**

II. Torsades de pointes
  -Correct underlying cause and consider discontinuing drugs that cause Torsades de pointes (quinidine, procainamide, disopyramide, moricizine, sotalol, ibutilide, bepridil, lidocaine, amiodarone, phenothiazines, tricyclic and tetracyclic antidepressants, vasopressin, imidazoles, pentamidine); correct hypokalemia and hypomagnesemia.
  -Magnesium sulfate (drug of choice) 1-4 gm IV bolus over 5-15 min or infuse 3-20 mg/min for 7-48h until QT interval <0.44 sec.
  -Isoproterenol (Isuprel) 2-20 µg/min (2 mg in 500 mL D5W, 4 µg/mL) **OR**
  -Phenytoin (Dilantin) 100-300 mg IV given in 50 mg increments q5min.
  -Consider ventricular pacing and cardioversion.

III. Other antiarrhythmics
Class Ib
  -Lidocaine 50-100 mg IV, then 2-4 mg/min IV.
  -Mexiletine (Mexitil) 100-200 mg PO q8h, max 1200 mg/d.
  -Tocainide (Tonocard) loading 400-600 mg PO, then 400-600 mg PO q8-12h; max 1800 mg/d.
  -Phenytoin (Dilantin), loading dose 100-300 mg IV given as 50 mg in NS over 10 min IV q5min, then 100 mg IV q5min prn.

Class Ic
  -Flecainide (Tambocor) 50-100 mg PO q12h, max 400 mg/d.
  -Propafenone (Rythmol) 150-300 mg PO q8h, max 1200 mg/d.

Class III
  -Amiodarone (Cordarone) PO loading 400-1200 mg/d in divided doses x 5-14 days, then 200-400 mg PO qd **OR**
  150 mg slow IV over 10 min, then 1 mg/min IV infusion x 6 hours then 0.5 mg/min IV infusion thereafter.
  -Sotalol (Betapace) 40-80 mg PO bid, max 320 mg/d in 2 divided doses.
  -Bretylium 5-10 mg/kg IV over 5-10 min, then maintenance of 1-4 mg/min IV or repeat boluses 5-10 mg/kg IV q6-8h; infusion of 1-4 mg/min IV.
  Labs: SMA 12, Mg, calcium, CBC, cardiac enzymes, LFT's, ABG, drug levels, thyroid function test. ECG, electrophysiologic study.

Pericarditis

Labs: CBC, SMA 12, albumin, Viral serologies: Coxsackie A & B, measles, mumps, influenza, ASO titer, hepatitis surface antigen, ANA, rheumatoid factor, anti-myocardial antibody, PPD with candida, mumps. Cardiac enzymes q8h x 4, ESR, complement thyroid panel, PT/PTT, blood C&S X 2. ECG, echocardiogram, CXR PA & LAT.

Pericardiocentesis: Gram stain, C&S, Thayer-Martin culture for gonococcus, cell count & differential, cytology, glucose, protein, LDH, amylase, triglyceride, AFB, fungal, specific gravity, pH, LE prep, rheumatoid factor.

Nonpurulent pericarditis

-Aspirin 650 mg PO q4-6h (2-3 gm/d) **OR**

Indomethacin (Indocin) 25-75 mg PO tid **OR**

Ibuprofen 400 mg PO tid or qid

-Morphine 2-4 mg IV q10 min prn pain; narcotics should be used cautiously if possible tamponade or constriction-may cause hypotension **OR**

Meperidine 50-100 mg IV q4h prn pain and Promethazine (Phenergan) 25-75 mg IV q4h.

-Prednisone 40-60 mg PO qd.

Purulent pericarditis

-Nafcillin or Oxacillin 2 gm IV q4h **AND EITHER**

-Gentamicin or tobramycin 100-120 mg IV (1.5-2 mg/kg); then 80 mg (1.0-1.5 mg/kg) IV q8h (adjust in renal failure) **OR**

-Ceftizoxime 1-2 gm IV q8h.

-Vancomycin, 1 gm IV q12h, may be used in place of nafcillin or oxacillin.

Temporary Pacemakers

Temporary pacemakers: Placed acutely for life threatening conduction blocks and bradycardia.

Transvenous pacemakers: Inserted into the right heart via the subclavian, femoral vein, or jugular veins. The generator is attached to the leads.

External pacemakers: Place one paddle posteriorly between the scapulae, and the other on the sternum. An external pace maker is a temporary measure until a transvenous pacer can be inserted.

Indications:

Prophylactic: New right bundle branch block (RBBB) with left heart block (LHB), alternating bundle branch block (BBB), Mobitz type II, complete heart block.

Therapeutic: Symptomatic bradycardia unresponsive to medical therapy; heart rate <50 with symptoms; sequential pacing of atria and ventricles when hemodynamically compromised by AV dissociation.

Management of transvenous pacer problems:

-If the patient is unstable, place the external pacer paddles on and turn output up until capture occurs.

-If the pacer does not capture, turn the output to maximum voltage. If this measure fails, try turning the sensitivity up (lower threshold voltage). Change batteries or change units.

-Order daily portable CXR to rule out pneumothorax and check lead placement.

-Record daily threshold measurements

Permanent Pacemakers

General Considerations: Leads are placed transvenously either in the right ventricle, right atrium, or both. Leads are attached to a pulse generator that is sutured below the skin.

Five Position Pacemaker Code

Chamber Paced	Chamber Sensed	Response to Sensing	Programmable functions	Anti-tachycardia functions
Ventricle	Ventricle	Triggers	Programmable	Programm-able
Atrium	Atrium	Inhibits	Multiprogrammable	Shock
Double	Double	Double: T or I	Communicates	Double: P and S
O-none	O-none	O-none	Rate modulation	

Most pacemakers are VVI or DDD.

Indications for Permanent Pacemakers:
Complete heart block (regardless of symptoms).
Mobitz II if symptomatic BBB with or without symptoms (depending on patterns)
Sick Sinus Syndrome if symptomatic or if beta blocker or calcium blocker therapy is planned
Carotid sinus hypersensitivity if symptomatic.
Post pacemaker implantation:
Immediate and daily CXR should be ordered to rule out pneumothorax and evaluate lead position. Check wound condition daily.

References
Ryan TJ, et al: ACC/AHN Guidelines for management of patients with acute myocardial infarction. JACC 1996;28:1328-1419.
Stone GW. Influence of Acute myocardial infarction location on in-hospital and late outcome after primary percutaneous transluminal coronary angioplasty versus t-PA therapy. AM J Cardiol 1996; 78:19-25.
The GUSTO Investigators: An international randomized trial comparing four thrombolytic strategies for acute myocardial infarction. N Engl J Med 1993; 329: 673-682.
Ram CV. Management of hypertensive emergencies: changing therapeutic options. American Heart Journal. [JC:3bw] 122(1 Pt 2):356-63, 1991 Jul.
Alastair JJ, eta I. The management of chronic heart failure. N Engl J ME 1996; 335:490-498.
Phillipa, ST, Whismant, JP: Hypertension and the brain. Arch Intern Med 1992;152:938
Granger C.B., Hirsh J, et al: Activated Partial Thromboplastin time and outcome after thrombolysis for Acute Myocardial Infarction. Results from the GUSTO-1 trial. Circulation 1996; 93:870-878.
The Sixth Report of the Joint National Committee on Prevention, Detection, Evaluation, and Treatment of High Blood Pressure. Arch Intern med. 1997; 157:2413-2445.
An international randomized trial comparing thrombolytic strategies in acute myocardial infarction. The GUSTO Trial. NEJM 1993; 329:673-82.

Pulmonary Disorders

Thomas Vovan, MD

Orotracheal Intubation

Endotracheal Tube Size (interior diameter):
Women 7.0-9.0 mm
Men 8.0-10.0 mm

1. Prepare suction apparatus. Have Ambu bag and mask apparatus setup with 100% oxygen; and ensure that patient can be adequately bagged and suction apparatus is available.
2. If sedation and/or paralysis is required, consider rapid sequence induction as follows:
   A. Fentanyl (Sublimaze) 50 meg increments IV (1 meg/kg) with:
   B. Midazolam (Versed) 1 mg IV q2-3 min. max 0.1-0.15 mg/kg followed by:
   C. Succinylcholine (Anectine) 0.6-1.0 mg/kg, at appropriate intervals.
   D. These drugs may cause vomiting; therefore, cricoid cartilage pressure should be applied during intubation (Sellick maneuver).
3. Position the patient's head in sniffing position with head flexed at neck and extended. If necessary, elevate head with a small pillow.
4. Ventilate patient with bag mask apparatus and hyperoxygenate with 100% oxygen.
5. Hold laryngoscope handle with left hand, and use right hand to open patient s mouth. Insert blade along the right side of mouth to the base of tongue, and push the tongue to the left. If using curved blade, advance to the vallecula (superior to epiglottis), and lift anteriorly, being careful not to exert pressure on the teeth. If using a straight blade, place beneath the epiglottis and lift anteriorly.
6. Place endotracheal tube (ETT) into right corner of mouth and pass it through the vocal cords; stop just after the cuff disappears behind vocal cords. If unsuccessful after 30 seconds, stop and resume bag and mask ventilation before re-attempting. Use a stilette to maintain the shape of the ETT (a hockey stick shape may be helpful); remove stillette after intubation. Application of lubricant jelly at endotracheal tube balloon facilitates passage through the vocal cords.
7. Inflate cuff with syringe keeping cuff pressure <20 cm H20 and attach the tube to an Ambu bag or ventilator. Confirm bilateral, equal expansion of the chest and equal bilateral breath sounds. Auscultate abdomen to confirm that the ETT is not in the esophagus. If there is any question about proper ETT location, repeat laryngoscopy with tube in place to be sure it is endotracheal; remove tube immediately if there is any doubt about proper location. Secure the tube with tape and note centimeter mark at the mouth. Suction the oropharynx and trachea.
8. Confirm proper tube placement with a chest X-ray (tip of ETT should be between the carina and thoracic inlet, or level with the top of the aortic notch).

Nasotracheal Intubation

Nasotracheal intubation is the preferred method if prolonged intubation is anticipated (increased patient comfort). Intubation will be facilitated if patient is awake and spontaneously breathing. There is an increased incidence of sinusitis with nasotracheal intubation.

1. Spray nasal passage with a vasoconstrictor such as cocaine 4% or phenylephrine 0.25% (Neo-Synephrine) may be used. If sedation is required before nasotracheal intubation, administer midazolam (Versed) 0.05-0.1 mg/kg IV push. Lubricate nasal airway with lidocaine ointment. Tube Size:
   Women 7.0mm tube
   Men 8.0, 9.0-mm tube
2. Place the nasotracheal tube into the nasal passage and guide it into nasopharynx along a U-shaped path. Monitor breath sounds by listening and feeling the end of tube. As the tube enters the oropharynx, gradually guide the tube downward. If the breath sounds stop, withdraw the tube 1-2 cm until breath sounds are heard again. Reposition the tube, and, if necessary, extend the head and advance. If difficulty is encountered, perform direct laryngoscopy and insert tube under direct visualization, or use Magill forceps.
3. Successful intubation occurs when the tube passes through the cords; a cough may occur and breath sounds will reach maximum intensity if the tube is correctly positioned. Confirm correct placement by checking for bilateral breath sounds and expansion of chest.
4. Confirm proper tube placement with chest x-ray.

Respiratory Failure and Ventilator Management

I. **Indications for Ventilatory Support**. Respirations >35, vital capacity <15 mL/kg, negative inspiratory force < -25, pO2 <60 on 50% 02. pH <7.2, pCO2 > 55, severe, progressive, symptomatic hypercapnia and/or hypoxia, severe metabolic acidosis.

II. **Initiation of Ventilator Support**
   A. **Intubation**
      1. **Prepare suction apparatus**, laryngoscope, endotracheal tube (No. 8 if possible); clear airway and place oral airway, hyperventilate with bag and mask attached to high flow oxygen.
      2. **Midazolam (Versed)** 1-2 mg IV boluses until sedated.
      3. **Intubate**, inflate cuff, ventilate with bag, auscultate chest, and suction trachea.
   B. **Initial Orders**
      1. **Assist control (AC)** 8-14 breaths/min, tidal volume = 750 mL (10-12 mL/kg ideal body weight), FiO2 = 100%, PEEP = 3-5 cm H20, Set rate so that minute ventilation (VE) is approximately 10 L/min.. Alternatively, use intermittent mandatory ventilation (IMV) mode with same tidal volume and rate to achieve near-total ventilatory support. Consider incorporating pressure support in addition to IMV at 5-15 cm H20.
      2. **ABG** should be obtained. Check ABG for adequate ventilation and oxygenation. If PO2 is adequate and Pulse Oximetry >98% then one

can titrate FiO2 to a safe level (FIO2<60%) by observing the saturation via pulse oximetry. Repeat ABG when target FiO2 is reached.

3. **Chest x-ray for tube placement**, measure cuff pressure q8h (maintain <20 mm Hg), pulse oximeter, arterial line, and/or monitor end tidal CO2. Maintain oxygen saturation >90-95%.

Ventilator Management

A. **Decreased Minute Ventilation.** Evaluate patient and rule out complications (endotracheal tube malposition, cuff leak, excessive secretions, bronchospasms, pneumothorax, worsening pulmonary disease, sedative drugs, pulmonary infection). Readjust ventilator rate to maintain mechanically assisted minute ventilation of 10 L/min. If peak airway pressure (AWP) is >45 cm H20, decrease tidal volume to 7-8 L/kg (with increase in rate if necessary), or decrease ventilator flow rate.

B. **Arterial Saturation >94% and pO$_2$ >100**, reduce FIO$_2$ (each 1%decrease in FIO$_2$ reduces pO$_2$ bye7 mm Hg); once FIO2 is <60%,PEEP may be reduced by increments of 2 cm H20 until PEEP = 3-5cm H20. Maintain O$_2$ saturation of >90% (pO$_2$ >60).

C. **Arterial saturation <90% and pO$_2$ <60**, increase FIO$_2$ up to 60-100%, then consider increasing PEEP by increments of 3-5 cm H20 (PEEP >10 requires a PA catheter). Add additional PEEP until oxygenation is adequate with an FIO$_2$ of <60%. Consider differential diagnosis of acute respiratory failure to find the cause of hypoxemia.

D. **Excessively low pH,** (pH <7.33 because of respiratory acidosis/hypercapnia): Increase rate and/or tidal volume. Keep peak airway pressure <40-50 cm H20 if possible.

E. **Excessively high pH** (>7.48 because of respiratory alkalosis/hypocapnia): Reduce rate and/or tidal volume to less. If patient is breathing rapidly above ventilator rate, consider sedation.

F. **Patient "Fighting Ventilator":** Consider IMV or SIMV mode, or add sedation with or without paralysis (exclude complications or other causes of agitation). Paralytic agents should not be used without concurrent amnesia and/or sedation.

G. **Sedation**
   1. **Diazepam (Valium)** 2-5 mg slow IV q2h pm agitation OR
   2. **Midazolam (Versed)** 0.05 mg/kg IVP x1, then 0.02-0.1 mg/kg/hr IV infusion. Titrate in increments of 25-50%.
   3. **Lorazepam (Ativan)** 1-2 mg IV ql-2h pm sedation or 0.05 mg/kg IVP x1, then 0.025-0.2 mg/kg/hr IV infusion. Titrate in increments of 25-50%.
   4. **Morphine Sulfate** 2-5 mg IV q1h or 0.03-0.05 mg/kg/h IV infusion (100 mg in 250 mL D5W) titrated OR
   5. **Propofol (Diprivan)**: 50 mcg/kg bolus over 5 min. then 5-50 mcg/kg/min. Titrate in increments of 5 mcg/kg/min.

H. **Paralysis** (with simultaneous amnesia):
   1. **Vecuronium (Norcuron)** 0.1 mg/kg IV, then 0.06 mg/kg/h IV infusion; intermediate acting, maximum neuromuscular blockade within 3-5 min. Half life 60 min OR

2. **Cisatracurium (Nimbex)** 0.15 mg/kg IV, then 0.3 mcg/kg/min IV infusion, titrate between 0.5-10 mcg/kg/min. Intermediate acting with half-life of 25 minutes. Plasma Cleared. Drug of choice for patient with renal/liver impairment OR

3. **Pancuronium (Pavulon)** 0.08 mg/kg W, then 0.03 mg/kg/h infusion. Long acting, half life 110 minutes, may cause tachycardia and/or hypertension OR

4. **Atracurium (Tracrium)** 0.5 mg/kg IV, then 0.3-0.6 mg/kg/h infusion, short acting, Half life 20 minutes. Histamine releasing properties may cause bronchospasm and/or hypotension.

f. **Monitor level of paralysis** with a peripheral nerve stimulator. Adjust neuromuscular blocker dosage to achieve a "train-of-four" (TOF) of 90-95%; if inverse ratio ventilation is being used, maintain TOF at 100%. Paralytic agents may cause prolonged muscle weakness in ICU patients, particularly when combined with steroids.

I. **Loss at Tidal Volume:** If a difference between the tidal volume setting and the delivered volume occurs, check for a leak in the ventilator or inspiratory line. Check for a poor seal between the endotracheal tube cuff or malposition of the cuff in the subglottic area. If a chest tube is present, check for air leak.

J. **High Peak pressure:** If Peak pressure is > 40-50 acutely consider causes (i.e Bronchospasm, Secretion, Pneunothorax, ARDS, Agitation, "Bucking the Ventilator"). First Suction patient and auscultate lungs. Obtain Chest radiograph if pneumothorax, pneumonia or ARDS is suspected. Check '"plateau pressure" if obtainable to differentiate airway resistance from compliance causes.

K. **Weaning parameters** should be obtained when weaning is being considered.

Inverse Ratio Ventilation

1. Indications: ARDS physiology, pAO_2 <60 mm Hg, FIO_2 >0.6, peak airway pressure >45 cm H_2O, or PEEP > 15 cm H_2O. This type of ventilatory support requires heavy sedation and respiratory muscle relaxation.

2. Set oxygen concentration (FIO_2) at 1.0; inspiratory pressure at ½ to 2/3 of the peak airway pressure on standard ventilation; set the inspiration: expiration ratio at 1: 1; set rate at <15 breaths/min. Maintain tidal volume by adjusting inspiratory pressures. Monitor auto-PEEP level.

3. Monitor PaO_2, oxygen saturation (by pulse oximetry), $PaCO_2$, end tidal PCO_2, PEEP, mean airway pressure, heart rate, blood pressure, SVO_2, and cardiac output.

4. It SaO_2 remains <0.9, consider increasing I:E ratio (2:1, 3:1), but generally attempt to keep I:E ratio < 2:1. If SaO_2 remains <0.9, increase PEEP or return to conventional mode. If $PaCO_2$ is excessively high, evaluate tracings to determine appropriate management. If hypotension develops, rule out tension pneumothorax, administer intravascular volume or pressor agents, decrease I:E ratio or rerum to conventional ventilation mode.

Ventilator Weaning

I. Ventilator Weaning Parameters
  A. Patient alert and rested
  B. PaO_2 >70 mm Hg on FiO_2 <50%
  C. $PaCO_2$ <50 mm Hg; pH >7.25
  D. Negative Inspiratory Force (NIF) more negative than -20 cm H_2O
  E. Vital Capacity >10-15 mL/kg (800-1000 mL)
  F. Minute Ventilation (VE) <10 L/min; respirations <24 breaths per min (at steady state)
  G. Maximal voluntary minute (MVV) ventilation doubles that of resting minute ventilation (VE).
  H. PEEP <5 cm H_2O
  I. Tidal volume 5-8 mL/kg
  J. Respiratory rate to tidal volume ratio <105
  K. No chest wall or cardiovascular instability or excessive secretions
  L. Neurologically capable of guarding airway.

II. Weaning Protocols
  A. Weaning is considered when patient medical condition (i.e. cardiac, pulmonary) status has stabilized. Successful wean from the ventilator requires constant attention to overall patient and ventilator interaction.
  B. **Indications for Termination at Weaning Trial**
    1. PaO_2 falls below 55 mmHg
    2. Acute hypercapnia
    3. Deterioration of vital signs or clinical status (arrhythmia)
  C. **Weaning trials** should start early in the morning to avoid extubation at night when staffing is sparse.
  D. **Rapid T-tube Weaning Method for Short-term (<7 days) Ventilator Patients without COPD**
    1. **Obtain baseline respiratory rate, pulse, blood pressure** and arterial blood gases or oximetry. Discontinue sedation, have well rested patient sit in bed or chair. Provide bronchodilators, and suctioning if needed.
    2. **Attach endotracheal tube** to a T-tube with FiO_2> 10% greater than previous level. Set T-tube flow-by rate to exceed peak inspiratory flow.
    3. **Patients who are tried on T-tube trial** should be observed closely for signs of deterioration. After initial 15 minute interval of spontaneous ventilation, resume mechanical ventilation and check oxygen saturation or draw an arterial blood gas sample.
    4. **If the 30 minute blood gas is acceptable**, a 60 minute interval may be attempted. After each interval the patient is placed back on the ventilator for an equal amount of time.
    5. **If the 60 minute interval blood gas is acceptable** and the patient is without dyspnea, and if blood gases are acceptable, extubation may be considered.
  E. **Pressure Support Ventilation Weaning Method**
    1. **Pressure support ventilation is initiated at 5-25 cm H_2O.** Set level to maintain the spontaneous tidal volume at 7-15 mL/kg.
    2. **Gradually decrease the level of pressure support** ventilation in increments of 3-5 cm H_2O according to the ability of the patient to maintain satisfactory minute ventilation.

     3. Extubation can be considered at a pressure support ventilation level of 5 cm H20 and patient can maintain stable respiratory status and blood gasses.

F. Intermittent Mandatory Ventilation (IMV) Weaning Method

  1. Obtain baseline vital signs, and draw baseline arterial blood gases or pulse oximetry. Discontinue sedation; consider adding pressure support of 10-15 cm H20 to provide support for those breaths that are not assisted.

  2. Change the ventilator from assist control to IMV mode; or if already on IMV mode, decrease the rate as follows:

    a. Patients with no underlying lung disease and on ventilator for a brief period (≤**1** week).

      (1) Decrease IMV rate at 30 min interval by 1-3 breath per min at each step, starting at rate of 8-10 until a rate for zero is reached.

      (2) If each step is tolerated and ABG is adequate (pH> 7.3-7.35), extubation may be considered.

      (3) Alternatively: The patient may be watched on minimal support (ie. Pressure support with CPAP) after IMV rate of zero is reached, then if no deterioration is noted then extubate.

    b. Patients with COPD or Prolonged ventilator support (>1 week)

      (1) Begin with IMV at frequency of 8 breath/minute, with tidal volume of 10 ml/kg, with an FiO2 10% greater than previous setting. Check end tidal CO2.

      (2) ABG should be drawn at 30 and 60 minute interval to check for adequate ventilation and oxygenation. If patient and/or blood gas deteriorate during weaning trial then return to previous stable setting.

      (3) Decrease IMV rate in increment of 1-2 breath per hour if the patient clinical status and blood gases stay stable. Check ABG and saturation one half hour after a new rate is set.

      (4) If the patient tolerates an IMV rate of zero, decrease the pressure to support in increment of 2-5 cm H20/hour until a pressure support of 5 cm H20 is reached.

      (5) Observe the patient for an additional 24 hours on minimal support before extubation.

  3. Causes of Inability to Wean Patients from Ventilators: Bronchospasm, active pulmonary infection, secretions, small endotracheal tube, weakness of respiratory muscle, low cardiac output.

Pulmonary Embolism

Pulmonary embolism should be considered in any patient with acute respiratory symptoms. Nearly three-quarters of a million episodes of pulmonary embolism occur each year. Pulmonary embolism is usually caused by thrombus formation is in the larger veins above the knee.

I. Risk factors for pulmonary embolism
   A. **Venous stasis.** Prolonged immobilization, hip surgery, stroke, myocardial infarction, heart failure, obesity, varicose veins, anesthesia, age >65 years old.
   B. **Endothelial injury.** Surgery, trauma, central venous access catheters, pacemaker wires, previous thromboembolic event.
   C. **Hypercoagulable state.** Malignant disease, high estrogen level (oral contraceptives).
   D. **Hematologic disorders.** Polycythemia, leukocytosis, thrombocytosis, antithrombin III deficiency, protein C deficiency, protein S deficiency, antiphospholipid syndrome, inflammatory bowel disease, factor 5 Leiden defect.

II. Diagnosis of pulmonary embolism
   A. Pulmonary embolism should suspected in any patient with new cardiopulmonary symptoms or signs and significant risk factors. If no other satisfactory explanation can be found in a patient with findings suggestive of pulmonary embolism, the workup for PE must be pursued to completion.
   B. **Signs and symptoms of pulmonary embolism.** Pleuritic chest pain, unexplained shortness of breath, tachycardia, hypoxemia, hypotension, hemoptysis, cough, syncope.
   C. The classic triad of dyspnea, chest pain, and hemoptysis is seen in only 20% of patients. The majority of patients have only a few subtle symptoms or are asymptomatic.
   D. Patients with massive pulmonary emboli may experience sudden onset of precordial pain, dyspnea, syncope, or shock. Other findings include distended neck veins, cyanosis, diaphoresis, pre-cordial heave, loud P2, right ventricular S3, or murmur of tricuspid insufficiency.
   E. A deep venous thrombosis may be indicated by an edematous limb with an erythrocyanotic appearance, dilated superficial veins, and elevated skin temperature.

Frequency of Symptoms and Signs in Pulmonary Embolism

Symptoms	Frequency (%)	Signs	Frequency (%)
Dyspnea	84	Tachypnea (>16/min)	92
Pleuritic chest pain	74	Rales	58
Apprehension	59	Accentuated S2	53
Cough	53	Tachycardia	44
Hemoptysis	30	Fever (>37.8°C)	43
Sweating	27	Diaphoresis	36
Non-pleuritic chest pain	14	S3 or S4 gallop	34
Syncope		Thrombophlebitis	32

Conditions That Can Cause Acute Respiratory Symptoms

Acute bronchitis	Pericarditis
Acute myocardial infarction	Pneumonia
Asthma	Pneumothorax
Cardiogenic shock	Pulmonary edema
Congestive heart failure	Pulmonary embolism
Exacerbation of chronic obstructive pulmonary disease	Septic shock

---

III. Diagnostic evaluation

A. **Chest radiographs** are nonspecific and insensitive, and findings are normal in up to 40 percent of patients with pulmonary embolism. Abnormalities may include an elevated hemidiaphragm, focal infiltrates, atelectasis, and small pleural effusions.

B. **Electrocardiography** is nonspecific and often normal. The most common abnormality is sinus tachycardia. ST-segment or T-wave changes are also common findings. Occasionally, acute right ventricular strain causes tall peaked P waves in lead II, right axis deviation, right bundle branch block, or atrial fibrillation.

C. **Blood gas studies**

1. There is no level of arterial oxygen that can rule out pulmonary embolism. Most patients with pulmonary embolism have a normal arterial oxygen. Impaired gas exchange is best assessed by using the room air, alveolar-to-arterial (A-a) oxygen gradient:

A-a oxygen gradient = $147 - [\text{measured } pAO_2 + (PCO_2/(0.8)]$

2. A normal gradient should be no higher than 10 plus one tenth of the patient's age.

3. A normal A-a oxygen gradient is seen in 5-15% of patients with pulmonary emboli but is inconsistent with massive pulmonary embolism and hypotension. An elevated gradient is nonspecific and may be produced by almost any pulmonary disease.

D. **Ventilation-perfusion scan**

1. **Normal/near normal or high probability V/Q scans** are reasonably diagnostic. Patients with a clearly normal perfusion scan do not have a pulmonary embolism, and less than 5 percent of patients with near-normal scan have a pulmonary embolism. A high-probability scan has a 90 percent probability of a pulmonary embolism.

2. **A low-probability V/Q scan** can exclude the diagnosis of pulmonary embolism only if the patient has a clinically low probability of pulmonary embolism.

3. **Intermediate V/Q scans** are not diagnostic and usually indicate the need for further diagnostic testing. One-third of patients with intermediate scans have a pulmonary embolism.

E. **Venous imaging**

1. If the V/Q scan is nondiagnostic, a workup for deep venous thrombosis (DVT) should be pursued using duplex ultrasound. The identification of DVT in a patient with signs and symptoms suggesting pulmonary embolism proves the diagnosis of pulmonary embolism. A deep venous thrombosis can be found in 80% of cases of pulmonary emboli.

2. Inability to demonstrate the existence of a DVT does not significantly lower the likelihood of pulmonary embolism because clinically asymptomatic DVT may not be detectable.
3. Patients with a nondiagnostic V/Q scan and no demonstrable site of DVT should proceed to pulmonary angiography.

F. **Angiography**
1. Contrast pulmonary arteriography is the "gold standard" for the diagnosis of pulmonary embolism. False-negative results occur in 2-10% of patients. False-positive results are extremely rare.
2. Angiography carries a low risk of complications (minor 5%, major nonfatal 1%, fatal 0.5%).

IV. **Management of acute pulmonary embolism in stable patients**

A. **Oxygen** should be initiated for all patients.

B. **Heparin anticoagulation**
1. In the absence of specific contraindications, heparin therapy should be started as soon as the diagnosis of pulmonary embolism is suspected. Full dose heparin can be given immediately after major surgery.
2. **Heparin administration.** 80 U/kg IVP, then 18 U/kg/h IV infusion. Obtain aPTT in 6 hours, and adjust dosage based on the table below to maintain the aPTT between 60-85 seconds.

Heparin Maintenance Dose Adjustment				
aPTT's	Bolus Dose	Stop infusion (min)	Rate Change, mL/h*	Repeat aPTT
<50	5000 U	0	+3 (increase by 150 U/h)	6 h
50-59	0	0	+2 (increase by 100 U/h)	6 h
60-85	0	0	0 (no change)	next AM
86-95	0	0	-1 (decrease by 50 U/h)	next AM
96-120	0	30	-2 (decrease by 100 U/h)	6 h
>120	0	60	-3 (decrease by 150 U/h)	6 h
*50 U/mL				

3. Platelet count should be monitored during heparin therapy; thrombocytopenia develops in up to 5%. Heparin may rarely induce hyperkalemia, which resolves spontaneously upon discontinuation.
4. **Warfarin (Coumadin)** may be started as soon as the diagnosis of pulmonary embolism is confirmed and heparin has been initiated. Starting dose is 10 mg PO qd for 3 days. The dose is then adjusted to

keep the International Normalized Ratio (INR) at 2.0 to 3.0. The typical dosage is 2.0-7.5 mg PO qd.

5. Heparin and warfarin regimens are overlapped for 3 to 5 days before heparin is discontinued.

6. Therapy with warfarin is generally continued for 6 months. In patients with an ongoing risk factor or following a second episode of DVT, lifelong anticoagulation with warfarin may be necessary.

7. **Low-molecular-weight heparin (LMWH)**. LMWH is as effective as unfractionated heparin for DVT or uncomplicated pulmonary embolism. It does not require dosage adjustment and may allow for earlier hospital discharge. LMWH is given subcutaneously. Enoxaparin (Lovenox) 1 mg/kg SQ q12h.

V. Management of acute pulmonary embolism in unstable patients

A. Patients with pulmonary embolism who have severe hypoxemia or any degree of hypotension are considered to be in unstable condition.

B. Heparin and oxygen should be started immediately.

C. Fluid and pharmacologic management

1. In acute cor pulmonale, gentle pharmacologic preload reduction with furosemide unloads the congested pulmonary circuit and reduces right ventricular pressures.

2. Hydralazine, isoproterenol, or norepinephrine may be required. Pulmonary artery pressure monitoring may be helpful.

D. Thrombolysis

1. Unstable patients (systolic <90 mmHg) with proven pulmonary embolism require immediate clot lysis by thrombolytic therapy.

2. Tissue plasminogen activator (Activase) is recommended because it is the fastest-acting thrombolytic agent.

3. **Contraindications to thrombolytics**

   a. **Absolute contraindications.** Active bleeding, cerebrovascular accident or surgery within the past 2 months, intracranial neoplasms.

   b. **Relative contraindications.** Recent gastrointestinal bleeding, uncontrolled hypertension, recent trauma (cardiopulmonary resuscitation), pregnancy.

4. **Alteplase (tPA, Activase).** 100 mg by peripheral IV infusion over 2 hr.

5. **Streptokinase (Kabikinase, Streptase).** The period required for clot lysis is substantially longer with streptokinase than with tissue plasminogen activator. 250,000 IU by peripheral IV infusion over 30 min, then 100,000 IU/hr IV for 24 hr.

6. Heparin therapy should be initiated after cessation of the thrombolytic infusion. Heparin is started without a loading dose when the activated partial thromboplastin time is 1.5 times control rate at 18 U/kg/hr.

VI. Emergency thoracotomy

A. Emergency surgical removal of embolized thrombus is reserved for instances when there is an absolute contraindication to thrombolysis or when the patient's condition has failed to improve after thrombolysis.

B. Cardiac arrest from pulmonary embolism is an indication for immediate thoracotomy. §

Asthma

Asthma is a lung disease characterized by reversible airway obstruction, airway inflammation, and increased airway responsiveness. Asthma affects about 5% of the population and accounts for about 5,000 deaths a year. Asthma is related to hereditary and environmental factors, such as allergies, irritants, and viral infections.

I. Pathophysiology

A. Allergies are found in more than one half of adults and children with asthma. However, asthma with a late onset (ie, in persons over 40 years old) is more likely to be "intrinsic" or nonallergic and is often severe and steroid-dependent. An allergic response to microscopic house dust mites is responsible for the development of asthma in many patients. Infection with respiratory syncytial virus in infancy is associated with subsequent development of asthma.

B. Asthmatic inflammatory disease can be quite destructive; over time partially irreversible airway obstruction may develop.

II. Steps in asthma management

A. Beta-agonists are prescribed initially for most patients, and they are used on an "as-needed" basis. Inhaled corticosteroids are recommended for patients with asthma unless their symptoms are mild and occasional.

B. Nonsteroidal anti-inflammatory drugs such as inhaled cromolyn (Intal) are alternatives to inhaled corticosteroids or an additional medication for difficult cases. Theophylline is a third-line therapy and is an option for nocturnal asthma.

III. Factors affecting response to therapy

A. **Allergies** contribute to asthma in many patients, and desensitization with allergy shots is effective in selected patients.

B. **Environmental irritants.** Exposure to second-hand tobacco smoke, perfume, room deodorizers, cooking odors, household cleaning products, and outdoor air pollutants (ozone and sulfur dioxide) should be prevented. Gastroesophageal reflux may exacerbate asthma by stimulating parasympathetic output.

C. **Viral infections** often trigger asthma exacerbations; early aggressive treatment of asthma exacerbations lessens the severity of the attack.

IV. Treatment of mild asthma

A. Asthma is considered mild if cough and wheezing occur no more than 1-2 times a week.

B. **Primary therapy** consists of as-needed use of inhaled beta agonists bronchodilators for occasional asthma attacks.

C. Albuterol (Ventolin) MDI, 2-4 puffs as needed or powder 200 mcg/capsule inhaled as needed.

D. Pirbuterol (Maxair) MDI, 2-4 puffs as needed.

E. Bitolterol (Tornalate) MDI, 2-4 puffs as needed.

F. Fenoterol (Berotec) MDI, 2-4 puffs as needed.

G. Salmeterol (Serevent) is a long-acting agent beta-agonist; 2 puffs bid. It is helpful for patients with nocturnal symptoms, and it should be used in moderate to severe asthma, combined with an inhaled steroid. Salmeterol should not be used in acute asthma.

H. Avoidance of dust and animals and the use of pillow and mattress covers are also recommended.

    I. Inhaled steroids should be started when patients need large daily doses of beta-agonists for symptomatic relief.

V. Treatment of moderate asthma

  A. Asthma is considered moderate if cough and wheezing occur more than 2 times a week or if there is exercise intolerance or nocturnal asthma.

  B. First-line therapy consists of frequent bronchodilator therapy "as needed" combined with an inhaled corticosteroid.

  C. Inhaled corticosteroids

    1. Asthma is an inflammatory process. All patients requiring a beta agonist more than occasionally should be treated with an inhaled corticosteroid agent. Steroids have disease-modifying activity, rather than simply promoting symptom control.

    2. Side effects include upper airway irritation, oropharyngeal Candida, and dysphonia.

      a. Beclomethasone (Beclovent, Vanceril, Vanceril DS) MDI, 4 puffs bid [42, 84 µg/puff].

      b. Triamcinolone (Azmacort) MDI, 4 puffs bid [100 µg/puff].

      c. Flunisolide (Aerobid) MDI, 4 puffs bid [250 µg/puff].

      d. Fluticasone (Flovent) MDI, 4 puffs bid [44, 110, 220 µg/puff].

      e. Budesonide (Pulmicort) dry powder inhaler, 4 puffs bid [200 µg/puff].

  D. Mast cell stabilizers

    1. Mast cell stabilizers, such as cromolyn (Intal), dampen the inflammatory response. They are better for maintaining good control in asthma rather than improving uncontrolled attacks.

    2. These agents are an alternative to corticosteroid inhalers or a safe addition to the regimen in a difficult case. They are useful in cases of allergic or exercise-induced asthma. These drugs are not as potent clinically as inhaled corticosteroids.

    3. Cromolyn (Intal), 2 puffs qid, or powder 20 mg/capsule inhaled qid, or 2 mL nebulized qid.

    4. Nedocromil (Tilade), 2 puffs tid-qid.

  E. Leukotriene blocking agents

    1. Leukotrienes are associated with asthma because they cause bronchoconstriction, stimulate mucus production, cause edema, and draw eosinophils into the airway.

    2. Inhaled steroids remain the anti-inflammatory drug of choice. However, leukotriene-blocking drugs may be useful in aspirin-sensitive asthmatics who are particularly likely to benefit from leukotriene blockers. They may be useful in patients who can not tolerate or require high doses of steroids.

    3. Montelukast (Singular) 10 mg PO qhs. No hepatotoxicity or drug interaction occurs.

    4. Zafirlukast (Accolate) is an oral leukotriene receptor antagonist; 20 mg bid. Churg-Strauss syndrome (eosinophilic vasculitis) has rarely been reported. Inhibition of warfarin metabolism may occur.

    5. Zileuton (Zyflo) is an oral lipoxygenase inhibitor; 600 mg qid. Reversible hepatitis develops in 2-4%; initial LFT monitoring is recommended. Inhibition of theophylline and warfarin metabolism may occur.

VI. Treatment of severe asthma

    A. Severe asthma is characterized by daily wheezing and/or a tendency for severe exacerbations.

    B. Maximal doses of inhaled bronchodilating agents plus aerosol corticosteroids should be used. When metered-dose inhalers are used in large doses (eg, 8 to 10 puffs per treatment), their effectiveness is comparable to that of nebulized therapy.

    C. Long-term, systemic corticosteroids

        1. The lowest effective dosage (alternate days when possible) should be used. Short-term oral therapy is the most effective method of treating refractory asthma, and it is more effective when instituted early.

        2. Prednisone 20 mg PO bid for 5-7 days, tapering over 7-14 days is seldom necessary except in patients who have been treated for more than 2 weeks.

        3. Some patients with severe asthma may require oral corticosteroids on a long-term basis. Doses taken on alternate days are preferred, and attempts should be made to find the minimum dose that is required for control. Long-term side effects include cataracts, osteoporosis, weight gain, skin fragility, fluid retention, growth suppression, exacerbation of diabetes, and suppression of the hypothalamic-pituitary-adrenal axis.

    D. Theophylline is a third-line therapy. The bronchodilating effects of theophylline are much weaker than those of beta agonists; however, it has mild anti-inflammatory activity and patient compliance is good with once- or twice-daily oral formulations. It still has a role in asthma therapy.

        1. Side effects include nausea, headache, insomnia, tremor, arrhythmias, and seizures. Serum levels are affected by cimetidine, ciprofloxacin, macrolides (erythromycin), and zileutin.

        2. Theophylline sustained release (Theo-Dur, Elixophyllin, Uniphyl) 100-400 mg PO bid [100, 200, 300, 450 mg]. Theo-24, 100-400 mg qd [100, 200, 300, 400 mg].

VII. Emergency treatment of asthma

    A. Albuterol (Ventolin) nebulized, 2.5 mg in 3 mL saline q20min initially, then q2-8h. Administer every 20 minutes for one hour, then clinically assess with a portable peak flow meter.

    B. If no improvement occurs within one hour, an intravenous corticosteroid should be administered. Methylprednisolone (Solu-Medrol) 80-125 mg IV q6h x 48-72 hours.

    C. Intravenous theophylline is of no additive benefit.

VIII. Adjunctive measures

    A. Portable peak flow meters are used for monitoring asthma status. Daily home peak flow meter readings should be maintained in the green zone (>80% of predicted peak flow). Yellow zone results (50-79%) indicate the need to augment baseline therapy. Peak flows in the red zone indicate the need for urgent medical treatment.

    B. Pulmonary function testing may be used to document airway disease.

    §

Chronic Obstructive Pulmonary Disease

Chronic obstructive pulmonary disease is the fourth leading cause of death in the United States. Emphysema and chronic bronchitis are the main disease states that comprise chronic obstructive pulmonary disease, although there is usually significant overlap between the two conditions.

I. Pathogenesis
   A. **Emphysema** is characterized by permanent enlargement of the alveolar air spaces with destruction of the alveolar walls.
   B. **Chronic bronchitis** is defined as chronic sputum production and variable degrees of airway obstruction for more than 3 months in each of 3 successive years.
   C. **Smoking** is the single overwhelming risk factor for the development of COPD. Pipe and cigar smokers are at intermediate risk for COPD.

II. Diagnosis of chronic obstructive pulmonary disease
   A. **Symptoms** are often insidious and may be manifest early by exercise intolerance. Later symptoms include wheezing, dyspnea, chronic cough, sputum production, recurrent pneumonias, and bronchitis.
   B. **Signs.** Wheezing, decreased air movement in the chest, hyperinflation, prolonged expiratory time, barrel chest, and supraclavicular retractions are characteristic.
   C. **Pulmonary function testing**
      1. Significant airway obstruction is present when the forced expiratory volume in 1 sec (FEV_1) is less than 80% of predicted, and the FEV_1/Forced Vital Capacity ratio is less than 70% of predicted.
      2. Hyperinflated lungs are indicated by an increased total lung capacity and residual volume and by loss of alveolar surface area and decreased diffusing capacity.

III. Management of chronic obstructive pulmonary disease
   A. **Smoking cessation** is effective in halting the progression of chronic obstructive pulmonary disease.
   B. **Anticholinergic agents**
      1. These drugs are first-line agents for COPD. Ipratropium may produce bronchodilation in patients who have no response to beta agonists and can reduce sputum volume without altering viscosity. It is not systemically absorbed and has minimal side effects. It should be used regularly with a beta agonist for most patients with COPD.
      2. **Ipratropium bromide (Atrovent)** 4-6 puffs qid or 2.5 mL (500 mcg) nebulized qid.
   C. **Beta agonists**
      1. **Beta2-adrenergic agonists** should be used for "as needed" treatment for symptom relief.
      2. **Side effects.** Tremor, nervousness, tachycardia, and hypokalemia in high doses.
      3. **Dosages**
         a. Albuterol (Ventolin) MDI, 2-4 puffs qid prn, or powder 200 mcg/capsule inhaled qid prn.
         b. Bitolterol (Tornalate) MDI, 2-4 puffs qid prn.
         c. Salmeterol (Serevent) MDI, 2 puffs bid; long-acting agent; useful for nocturnal symptoms; not effective for acute exacerbation because of slow onset of action.

D. Theophylline

1. Theophylline has utility in patients with significant side effects from high dose beta agonists (allowing the use of two drugs below their toxic levels) as well as in patients with nocturnal symptoms. It has been shown to improve airflows, decrease dyspnea, and improve collateral ventilation, arterial blood gases, exercise tolerance, respiratory muscle function, and mucociliary clearance.

2. It should be used after adequate doses of ipratropium and beta2-agonists have been tried. A dosage that yields a serum drug level ranging from 8 to 12 ug/mL is recommended. Evening dosing may control decreased nighttime airflows and improve morning respiratory symptoms.

3. Theophylline has significant toxicity and various conditions may acutely alter theophylline levels. Adverse drug interactions occur with ciprofloxacin, erythromycin, cimetidine, and zileuton.

4. **Dosage of long-acting theophylline.** 200-300 mg bid. Theophylline preparations with 24 hour action may be administered once a day in the early evening. Theo-24, 100-400 mg qd [100, 200, 300, 400 mg].

E. Corticosteroids

1. Corticosteroids produce a favorable response during acute COPD exacerbations, improving symptoms and reducing the length of hospitalization. Short courses of corticosteroids should be considered in patients with acute exacerbations who are unresponsive to aggressive inhaled bronchodilator therapy.

2. Long-term use of corticosteroids should be considered only in patients who have continued symptoms or severe airflow limitation despite maximal therapy with other agents. Only 20% to 30% of patients show objective benefits from long-term corticosteroid administration.

3. A closely monitored clinical trial should be used to select patients who might benefit from corticosteroid therapy. Oral and high-dose inhaled corticosteroids have both been used to assess long-term steroid response.

4. Only those patients with documented physiologic improvement following a steroid trial should be considered for long-term therapy, and the goal should be to achieve the lowest possible dose.

5. Aerosolized corticosteroids provide the benefits of oral corticosteroids with fewer side effects.
   Beclomethasone (Beclovent) MDI 2-5 puffs tid-qid.
   Triamcinolone (Azmacort) MDI 2-4 puffs bid-qid.
   Flunisolide (Aerobid, Aerobid-mint) MDI 2-4 puffs bid.
   Budesonide (Pulmicort) MDI 1-2 puffs bid.

6. Oral steroids are warranted in severe COPD. Prednisone 0.5-1.0 mg/kg or 40 mg may be given qAM. The dose should be tapered over 1-2 weeks following clinical improvement.

7. **Side effects of corticosteroids.** Cataracts, osteoporosis, sodium and water retention, hypokalemia, muscle weakness, aseptic necrosis of femoral and humeral heads, peptic ulcer disease, pancreatitis, endocrine and skin abnormalities, muscle wasting.

IV. Surgical treatment

A. Lung volume reduction surgery (LVRS) consists of surgical removal of an emphysematous bulla. This procedure can ameliorate symptoms and improve pulmonary function.

   B. Lung transplantation is reserved for those patients deemed unsuitable or too ill for LVRS. It is effective for severe emphysema.

V. Treatment of complications of COPD

A. Infection

1. Infection frequently causes bronchitis exacerbations and is associated with increased or purulent sputum, increased cough, chest congestion and discomfort, and increased dyspnea and wheezing. Chills and fever suggest pneumonia. Acute bacterial episodes tend to be seasonal, appearing more frequently in the winter.

2. **Gram Stain**

   a. Gram stain is a useful guide in the selection of an empiric antibiotic.

   b. The presence of more than 25 neutrophils and fewer than 10 epithelial cells per low-power field indicates that the specimen is sputum.

   c. The presence of bacteria on high-power examination of such a specimen is presumptive evidence of infection. Although patients with COPD may be colonized by Hemophilus influenzae and Streptococcus pneumoniae, these organisms should not be present in sufficient numbers to be seen on a Gram stain.

3. **Sputum culture and sensitivity** testing are generally not necessary but may be required if the patient is very ill or if the infection is hospital-acquired.

4. **A chest film** is helpful in ruling out pneumonia or other disorders.

5. The primary pathogens for COPD exacerbations include H. influenzae, parainfluenzae, S. pneumoniae, and Moraxella catarrhalis. Atypical organisms, such as Mycoplasma pneumoniae or Chlamydia, may be present. Other less common pathogens are staphylococci, Neisseria, Klebsiella, and Pseudomonas.

6. **Treatment of exacerbations of COPD**

   a. Treat 10-14 days.

   b. Trimethoprim/Sulfamethoxazole (Septra DS) 160/800 mg PO bid.

   c. Amoxicillin/clavulanate (Augmentin) 500 mg PO tid [250, 500 mg]; stable against beta lactamases; gastrointestinal side effects (diarrhea) are common.

   d. Cefuroxime axetil (Ceftin), 250-500 mg PO bid; good activity against primary pathogens; stable against beta lactamase.

   e. Cefixime (Suprax), 200 mg PO bid or 400 mg PO qd; stable against beta lactamase, lacks Staphylococcus aureus coverage.

   f. Doxycycline (Vibramycin), 100 mg bid; not affected by beta-lactamase, S pneumoniae resistance in 10-20%. Active against atypical pathogens.

   g. Azithromycin (Zithromax), 500 mg on day 1, then 250 mg PO qd; reserved for treatment of infections due to Mycoplasma, Chlamydia, Legionella species.

   h. Clarithromycin (Biaxin), 250-500 mg bid; moderate activity against H influenzae.

   i. Erythromycin, 250-500 mg qid; inexpensive; poor activity against H influenzae; raises theophylline levels.

   j. Levofloxacin (Levaquin) 500 mg PO qd. Broad spectrum coverage.

B. Hypoxemia
1. Hypoxemia adversely affects function and increases risk of death, and oxygen therapy is the only treatment documented to improve survival in patients with COPD.
2. Oxygen is usually delivered by nasal cannula at a flow rate sufficient to maintain an optimal oxygen saturation level. The flow rate should be increase by 1 liter per minute during exercise and sleep. §

Pleural Effusion

Labs: CBC, ABG, SMA 12, protein, albumin, amylase, rheumatoid factor, ANA, ESR. PT/PTT, UA. CXR PA & LAT repeat after thoracentesis, bilateral decubitus, ECG, ultrasound.

Pleural fluid Analysis:
> **Tube 1.** LDH, protein, amylase, triglyceride, glucose (10 mL).
> **Tube 2.** Gram stain, C&S, AFB, fungal C&S, wet mount (20-60 mL, heparinized).
> **Tube 3.** Cell count and differential (5-10 mL, EDTA).
> **Tube 4.** Sudan stain, LE prep, antigen tests for S pneumoniae, H influenza (25-50 mL, heparinized).
> **Syringe.** pH (2 mL collected anaerobically, heparinized on ice)
> **Bottle.** Cytology.

Differential Diagnosis		
Pleural Fluid Parameters	**Transudate**	**Exudate**
LDH (IU)	<200	>200
Pleural LDH/Serum LDH	<0.6	>0.6
Total Protein (g/dL)	<3.0	>3.0
Pleural Protein/Serum Protein	<0.5	>0.5

Differential Diagnosis of Transudates: Congestive heart failure, cirrhosis.
Differential Diagnosis of Exudates: Empyema, viral pleuritis, tuberculosis, neoplasm, uremia, drug reaction, asbestosis, sarcoidosis, collagen disease (lupus, rheumatoid disease), pancreatitis, subphrenic abscess.

References
Marcy TW, Manni JJ. Inverse ratio ventilation in ARDS. Rationale and implementation. Chest, 1991 100(2):404-504.
Kollef et al. The Acute Respiratory Distress syndrome. NEJM 1995,332(1):27-37
Amato et al. Effect of a protective-ventilation strategy on mortality in the ARDS. NEJM 1998,338(6)347-54

Yang KL; Tobin MJ. A prospective study of indexes predicting the outcome of teals of weaning from mechanical ventilation. NEJM, 1991 324(21): 1445-50.

Macintyre NR. Clinically available new strategies for mechanical ventilatory support. Chest, 1993, 104(2):500-5.

Tobin MJ. Mechanical Ventilation. NEJM, 1994, 330(15): 1056-61

Esteban A et al. A Comparison of four methods of weaning patients from mechanical ventilation. NEJM, 1995, 332 (6):345-350.

Hirsh J. et al: Management of deep vein thrombosis and pulmonary and pulmonary embolism. Circulation 1996, 93:2212-2245

The Columbus Investigators. Low-Molecular Weight Heparin in the Treatment of patients with venous thromboembolism. NEJM 1997, 337(10):657-662

McFadden ER Jr Gilbert IA. Asthma. NEJM. 1992, 327(27): 1928-37.

Trauma

Dan L. Serna, MD

Pneumothorax

I. Management of pneumothorax
  A. **Small primary spontaneous pneumothorax (<10-15%): (not associated with underlying pulmonary diseases). If the patient is not dyspneic**
    1. Observe for 4-8 hours and repeat a chest X-ray.
    2. If the pneumothorax does not increase in size and the patient remains asymptomatic, consider discharge home with instructions to rest and curtail all strenuous activities. Return if increase in dyspnea or recurrence of chest pain.
  B. **Secondary spontaneous pneumothorax (associated with underlying pulmonary pathology, most commonly emphysema) or primary spontaneous pneumothorax >15%, or if patient is symptomatic**
    1. Give high flow oxygen. A needle thoracotomy should be placed at the anterior, second intercostal space in the midclavicular line.
    2. Anesthetize and prep the area, then insert a 16-gauge needle with an internal catheter and a 60 mL syringe attached via a 3-way stopcock. Aspirate until no more air is aspirated. If no additional air can be aspirated, and the volume of aspirated air is <4 liters, occlude the catheter and observe for 4 hours.
    3. If symptoms abate and chest-x-ray does not show recurrence of the pneumothorax: the catheter can be removed, and the patient can be discharged home with instructions.
    4. If the aspirated air is >4 liters and additional air is aspirated without resistance, this represents an active bronchopleural fistula with continued air leak. Admission is required for insertion of a chest tube.
  C. **Traumatic Pneumothorax associated with a penetrating injury, hemothorax, mechanical ventilation, tension pneumothorax, or if pneumothorax does not resolve after needle aspiration:** Give high flow oxygen and insert a chest tube, along with aggressive hemodynamic and respiratory resuscitation as indicated. Do not delay the management of a tension pneumothorax until radiographic confirmation, insert needle thoracotomy or chest tube immediately.

II. Technique of Chest Tube Insertion
  A. Place patient in supine position, with involved side elevated 20 degrees; abduct arm at 90 degrees. The usual site is the fourth or fifth intercostal space, between the mid-axillary and anterior axillary line (drainage of air or free fluid). The point at which the anterior axillary fold meets the chest wall is a useful guide. Consult the chest radiograph for further guidance if time permits. Alternatively, the second or third intercostal space, in the mid-clavicular line, may be used for pneumothorax drainage alone (air only).
  B. Cleanse skin with Betadine iodine solution and drape the field. Determine the intrathoracic tube distance (lateral chest wall to the apices), and mark the length of tube with a clamp.

C. Infiltrate 1% lidocaine into the skin, subcutaneous tissues, intercostal muscles, periosteum, and pleura using a 25-gauge needle. Use a scalpel to make a transverse skin incision, 2 centimeters wide, located over the rib just inferior to the interspace where the tube will penetrate the chest wall.

D. Using a Kelly clamp to bluntly dissect a subcutaneous tunnel from the skin incision, extending just over the superior margin of the lower rib. Avoid the nerve, artery and vein located at the upper margin of the intercostal space.

E. Penetrate the pleura with the clamp, and open the pleura 1 centimeter.

F. With a gloved finger, explore the subcutaneous tunnel, and palpate the lung medially. Exclude possible abdominal penetration, and ensure correct location within pleural space; use finger to remove any local pleural adhesions.

G. Use the Kelly clamp to grasp the tip of the thoracostomy tube (36 F, internal diameter 12 mm), and direct it into the pleural space in a posterior, superior direction for pneumothorax evacuation. Direct tube inferiorly for pleural fluid removal. Guide the tube into the pleural space until the last hole is inside the pleural space and not inside the subcutaneous tissue.

H. Attach the tube to an underwater seal apparatus containing sterile normal saline, and adjust to 20 cm H_2O of negative pressure, or attach to suction if leak is severe. Suture the tube to the skin of the chest wall using O silk. Apply Vaseline gauze, 4 x 4 gauze sponges, and elastic tape. Obtain a chest X-ray to verify correct placement and evaluate reexpansion of lung.

Tension Pneumothorax

I. **Clinical Evaluation**

A. **Clinical Signs:** Severe hemodynamic and/or respiratory compromise; contralaterally deviated trachea; decreased or absent breath sounds and hyperresonance to percussion on the affected side; jugular venous distention, asymmetrical chest wall motion with respiration.

B. **Radiologic Signs:** Flattening or inversion of the ipsilateral hemidiaphragm; contralateral shifting of the mediastinum; flattening of the cardio-mediastinal contour and spreading of the ribs on the ipsilateral side.

II. **Acute Management**

A. A temporary large-bore IV catheter may be inserted into the ipsilateral pleural space, at the level of the second intercostal space at the mid-clavicular line until the chest tube is placed.

B. A chest tube should be placed emergently.

C. Draw blood for CBC, INR, PTT, type and cross-matching, Chem 7, Toxicology screen.

D. Send pleural fluid for hematocrit, amylase and pH (to rule out possible esophageal rupture).

E. **Indications for Cardiothoracic Exploration:** Severe or persistent hemodynamic instability despite aggressive fluid resuscitation, persistent active blood loss from chest tube, more than 200 cc/hr for 3 consecutive hours, or ≥ 1 1/2 L of acute blood loss after chest tube placement.

Cardiac Tamponade

I. General Considerations
A. Cardiac tamponade occurs most commonly secondary to penetrating injuries.
B. Beck's Triad: Venous pressure elevation, drop in the arterial pressure, muffled heart sounds.
C. Other Signs: Enlarged cardiac silhouette on CXR; signs and symptoms of hypovolemic shock; electromechanical dissociation (pulseless electrical activity), decreased voltage on ECG.
D. Kussmaul's sign is characterized by a rise in venous pressure with inspiration. Pulsus paradoxus or elevated venous pressure may be absent when associated with hypovolemia.

II. Management
A. Pericardiocentesis is indicated if patient is unresponsive to the usual resuscitation measures for hypovolemic shock, or if there is a high likelihood of injury to the myocardium or one of the great vessels.
B. All patients who have a positive pericardiocentesis (recovery of non-clotting blood) because of trauma, require an open thoracotomy with inspection of the myocardium and the great vessels.
C. Rule out other causes of cardiac tamponade such as pericarditis, penetration of central line through the vena cava, atrium, or ventricle, or infection.
D. Consider other causes of hemodynamic instability that may mimic cardiac tamponade (tension pneumothorax, massive pulmonary embolism, shock secondary to massive hemothorax).

Pericardiocentesis

I. General Considerations
A. If acute cardiac tamponade with hemodynamic instability is suspected, emergency pericardiocentesis should be performed; infusion of Ringer's lactate, crystalloid, colloid and/or blood may provide temporizing measures.

II. Management
A. Protect airway and administer oxygen. If patient can be stabilized, pericardiocentesis should be performed by a specialist in the operating room or catheter lab. The para-xiphoid approach is used for pericardiocentesis.
B. Place patient in supine position with chest elevated at 30-45 degrees, then cleanse and drape peri-xiphoid area. Infiltrate lidocaine 1% with epinephrine (if time permits) into skin and deep tissues.
C. Attach a long, large bore (12-18 cm, 16-18 gauge), short bevel cardiac needle to a 50 cc syringe with a 3-way stop cock. Use a alligator clip to attach a V-lead of the ECG to the metal of the needle.
D. Advance the needle just below costal margin, immediately to the left and inferior to the xiphoid process. Apply suction to the syringe while

advancing the needle slowly at a 45 degree horizontal angle towards the mid point of the left clavicle.

E. As the needle penetrates the pericardium, resistance will be felt, and a characteristic "popping" sensation will be noted.

F. Monitor the ECG for ST segment elevation (indicating ventricular heart muscle contact); or PR segment elevation (indicating atrial epicardial contact). After the needle comes in contact with the epicardiurn, withdraw the needle slightly. Ectopic ventricular beats are associated with cardiac penetration.

G. Aspirate as much blood as possible. Blood from the pericardial space usually will not clot. Blood, inadvertently, drawn from inside the ventricles or atrium usually will clot. If fluid is not obtained, redirect the needle more towards the head.

H. Stabilize the needle by attaching a hemostat or Kelly clamp.

I. Consider emergency thoracotomy to determine the cause of hemopericardium (especially if active bleeding). If the patient does not improve, consider other problems that may resemble tamponade, such as tension pneumothorax, pulmonary embolism, or shock secondary to massive hemothorax.

References

Committee on Trauma, American College of Surgeons: Early Care of the Injured Patient. Philadelphia, WB Sanders Co., 1982, pp 142-148.

Light RW. Management of Spontaneous Pneumothorax. Am. Rev. Res. Dis. 1993; 148, 1: 245-248.

Light RW. Pneumothorax. In: Light RW, ed. Pleural Diseases. Philadelphia; Lea & Farbiger, 1990; 237-62.

Hematologic Disorders

Thomas Vovan, MD

Transfusion Reactions

I. Acute Hemolytic Transfusion Reaction

A. Clinical Presentation: This rare reaction is most commonly associated with ABO incompatibility, and it is usually related to a clerical error. Early symptoms include sudden onset of anxiety, flushing, tachycardia, and hypotension. Chest and back pain, fever and dyspnea are common.

B. Life threatening manifestations include vascular collapse (shock), renal failure, bronchospasm, and disseminated intravascular coagulation.

C. Hemoglobinuria, and hemoglobinemia occurs because of intravascular red cell lysis.

D. A positive direct antiglobulin test (direct Coombs test) will be found after transfusion. The severity of reaction is usually related to the volume of RBC's infused.

E. Management

1. Discontinue transfusion and notify blood bank immediately. Send the unused donor blood and a sample of recipient's venous blood for retyping and repeat cross match including direct and indirect Coombs test.

2. Check urine analysis for free hemoglobin and check centrifuged plasma for pink coloration (indicating free hemoglobin).

3. Manage hypotension with normal saline or plasma expanders. Vasopressors may be used if volume replacement alone is inadequate to maintain blood pressure. Central venous monitoring may be necessary.

4. Maintain adequate renal perfusion with volume replacement. Mannitol and/or furosemide may be used to maintain urine output after adequate volume replacement has been achieved.

5. Monitor PT/PTT, platelets, fibrinogen, and fibrin degradation products for evidence of disseminated intravascular coagulation. Replace required clotting factors with fresh frozen plasma, platelets, and/or cryoprecipitate.

6. In rare circumstances, exchange transfusions have been performed for massive intravascular hemolysis.

II. Febrile Transfusion Reaction (nonhemolytic)

A. Clinical Presentation: This reaction occurs in 0.5-3% of transfusions, and is most commonly seen in patients receiving multiple transfusions. Chills develop followed by fever, usually during or within a few hours of transfusion. This reaction may be severe but is usually mild and self limited.

B. Management

1. Provide symptomatic and supportive care with acetaminophen and diphenhydramine. Meperidine 50 mg IV is useful in treating chills. A WBC filter should be used for the next transfusion.

2. More serious transfusion reactions must be excluded (eg, acute hemolytic reaction or bacterial contamination of donor blood).

III. Transfusion-related Noncardiogenic Pulmonary Edema

A. **Clinical Presentation** is characterized by sudden development of severe respiratory distress, associated with fever, chills, chest pain, and hypotension.

B. Chest radiograph demonstrates diffuse pulmonary edema. This reaction may be severe and life threatening but generally resolves within 48 hours.

C. **Management**
 1. Provide supportive measures for pulmonary edema and hypoxemia including mechanical ventilatory support and hemodynamic monitoring if needed.
 2. Diuretics are useful only if fluid overload is present.
 3. Use a WBC filter for next transfusion.

Disseminated Intravascular Coagulation

I. Clinical Manifestations

A. DIC is manifested by generalized ecchymosis and petechiae, bleeding from peripheral IV sites, central catheters, surgical wounds, and oozing from gums.

B. Gastrointestinal and urinary tract bleeding are frequently encountered. Grayish discoloration or cyanosis of the distal fingers, toes, or ears may occur because of intravascular thrombosis.

C. Large, sharply demarcated ecchymotic areas may be seen as a result of thrombosis of the dermal blood supply.

II. Diagnosis

A. Fibrin degradation products are the most sensitive screening test for DIC; however, no single laboratory parameter is diagnostic of DIC, and findings may be quite variable. Repeated testing of coagulation parameters may provide a kinetic assessment of the rate and degree of factor consumption or replacement.

B. **Peripheral Smear:** Evidence of microangiopathic hemolysis with schistocytes and thrombocytopenia are present. A persistently normal platelet count nearly excludes the diagnosis of acute DIC.

C. **Coagulation Studies:** INR, PTT, and thrombin time are generally prolonged. Fibrinogen levels are usually depleted (<150 mg/dL). Fibrin degradation products are elevated (>10 mg/dL). D-dimer is elevated (>0.5 mg/dL).

III. Management of Disseminated Intravascular Coagulation

A. The primary underlying precipitating condition (eg, sepsis) is treated. Reversal of the syndrome depends on the treatment of the underlying disorder.

B. Severe DIC with hypocoagulability may be treated with replacement of clotting factors; hypercoagulability is managed with inhibition of coagulation with heparin.

C. Severe hemorrhage and shock is managed with fluids and red blood cell transfusions.

D. **If the patient is at high risk of bleeding or actively bleeding with biochemical evidence of DIC:** Replace fibrinogen with 10 units of cryoprecipitate. Replace clotting factors with 2-4 units of fresh frozen plasma. Replace platelets with platelet phoresis.

E. **If factor replacement therapy is transfused,** fibrinogen and platelet levels should be obtained 30-60 minutes post-transfusion and every 4-6 hours thereafter to determine the efficacy of therapy. Each unit of platelets should increase the platelet count by 5000-10,000/mcL. Each unit of cryoprecipitate should increase fibrinogen level by 5-10 mg/dL.

F. **Heparin**
1. The use of heparin is controversial. Indications for heparin include evidence of fibrin deposition (i.e. dermal necrosis, acral ischemia, venous thromboembolism).
2. Heparin is used when the coagulopathy is believed to be secondary to a retained dead fetus, amniotic fluid embolus, giant hemangiomas, aortic aneurysm, solid tumors, or promyelocytic leukemia. Heparin is also used when clotting factors cannot be corrected with replacement therapy alone.
3. Heparin therapy is initiated at a relatively low dose (5-10 U/kg/hr) by continuous IV infusion without bolus. Coagulation parameters must then be followed to guide therapy. If desired increments of clotting factors do not occur, the heparin dose may be increased by 2.5 U/kg/hr until the desired effect is achieved.

Thrombolytic Associated Bleeding

I. **Clinical Presentation**: Post-fibrinolysis hemorrhage has varied presentations, including sudden neurologic deficit (intracranial bleeding), massive volume loss (as in GI bleeding), or gradual decline in hemoglobin without overt evidence of bleeding.

II. **Laboratory Evaluation**
A. Low fibrinogen (<100 mg/dL) and elevated fibrin degradation products confirm the presence of a lytic state.
B. Elevated thrombin time and PTT may suggest a persistent lytic state; however, both are prolonged in the presence of heparin.
C. Prolonged reptilase time identifies the persistent lytic state in the presence of heparin.
D. Depleted fibrinogen in the fibrinolytic state will be reflected by an elevated PTT, thrombin time, or reptilase time. The post-transfusion fibrinogen level is a useful indicator of response to replacement therapy.
E. The bleeding time, as an indicator of platelet function, may be a helpful guide to platelet replacement therapy if the patient has persistent bleeding despite factor replacement with cryoprecipitate, and fresh frozen plasma.

III. **Management**
A. Discontinue thrombolytics, aspirin, and heparin immediately, and consider protamine reversal of heparin and cryoprecipitate to replenish fibrinogen.
B. Place two large bore IV catheters for volume replacement. If possible, apply local pressure to bleeding sites.
C. Send blood specimens for INR/PTT, fibrinogen, and thrombin time. Check reptilase time if patient is also receiving heparin.
D. Patient's blood should be typed and crossed because urgent transfusion may be needed.

E. Transfusion
1. Cryoprecipitate (10 units over 10 minutes) should be transfused as a first-line measure to correct the lytic state. Transfusions may be repeated until the fibrinogen level is above 100 mg/dL or hemostasis is achieved.
2. Fresh frozen plasma transfusion is also important for replacement of factor VIII and V. If bleeding persists after cryoprecipitate and FFP replacement, check a bleeding time and consider platelet transfusion if bleeding time is greater than 9 minutes. If bleeding time is less than 9 minutes, then antifibrinolytic drugs may be warranted.

F. Antifibrinolytic Agents
1. Aminocaproic acid (EACA) inhibits the binding of plasmin to fibrin and plasminogen to fibrinogen. It is used when replacement of blood products are not sufficient to attain hemostasis; potential risk of serious thrombotic complications.
2. Loading dose: 5 g or 0.1 g/kg IV infused in 250 cc NS over 30-60 min, followed by continuous infusion at 0.5 to 1.0 g/h until bleeding is controlled. Use with caution in upper urinary tract bleeding because of the potential for obstruction. Contraindicated in DIC.

G. If bleeding is suspected on the basis of falling hemoglobin without overt evidence of blood loss: Occult sources must be considered, including the retroperitoneal space, thigh (often related to femoral venous or arterial puncture), bleeding into other body cavities (peritoneum, thorax).

References

Carr JM, McKinney M, McDonagh J: Diagnosis of Disseminated Intravascular Coagulation, Role of D-Dimer. Am J Clin Pathol 1989;91:280-287.

Feinstein DI: Treatment of Disseminated Intravascular Coagulation. Seminars in Thrombosis and Hemostasis. 1988;14:351-362.

Sane DC, Califf RM, Topol EJ, Stump DC, Mark DB, Greenberg CS: Bleeding during Thrombolytic Therapy for Acute Myocardial Infarction: Mechanisms and Management. Ann of Int Med. 1989;111:1010-1022.

Infectious Diseases

Feras Hawari, MD

Bacterial Meningitis

Meningitis is inflammation of the meninges, the membranes covering the brain and spinal cord, and it is characterized by pleocytosis of the cerebrospinal fluid.
I. Clinical Evaluation
  A. **The classic triad of fever, headache and stiff neck** occurs in more than 85% of patients with acute bacterial meningitis. The meningismus may be subtle, marked or accompanied by Kernig's and/or Brudzinski's signs (which occur in about 50%).
  B. **Vomiting** occurs in 35% of patients, seizures occur in 30% of patients, and cranial nerve palsies and focal cerebral signs occur in 20% of patients.
  C. **Lethargy or obtundation** may be the only insidious signs in elderly patients.
  D. **Examination of cerebrospinal fluid** values following lumbar puncture is necessary to make a definitive diagnosis of bacterial meningitis.

Cerebrospinal Fluid Values in Bacterial Meningitis	
Cerebrospinal fluid parameter	**Typical values**
Opening pressure	>180 mm H_2O
Leukocyte count	1,000 to 5,000 per mm^3
Percentage of neutrophils	$\geq 80\%$
Protein	100 to 500 mg per dL
Glucose	≤ 40 mg per dL
Gram stain	Positive in 60-90%
Culture	Positive in 70-85%

  E. Latex agglutination testing detects the antigens of common meningeal pathogens, such as Haemophilus influenzae type b, Streptococcus pneumoniae, Neisseria rneningitidis, Escherichia coli K1, and Streptococcus agalactiae. Results are available within 20 minutes. The overall sensitivity of the latex agglutination is 50-100%. The overall specificity is high. A positive latex agglutination test establishes the diagnosis of bacterial meningitis; however, a negative test never rules out bacterial meningitis.
  F. Polymerase chain reaction may be useful when Gram stain, bacterial antigen tests and cultures are negative.

II. Initial Approach to Management

A. A lumbar puncture must be performed to establish a definitive diagnosis. If results of the Gram stain or bacterial antigen tests of the cerebrospinal fluid are consistent with a diagnosis of bacterial meningitis, antimicrobial therapy should be initiated. However, if no etiologic agent can be identified, empiric antimicrobial therapy should be directed at the likely pathogen according to the age of the patient.

Empiric Treatment of Bacterial Meningitis		
Age	Common bacterial pathogens	Empiric antimicrobial therapy*
18 to 50 years	S. pneumoniae, N. meningitidis	Cefotaxime 2 gm IV q4h, or ceftriaxone 2 gm IV q12h) with or without ampicillin (2 gm IV q4h) if L. monocytogenes is suspected
Older than 50 years	S. pneumoniae, N. meningitidis, L. mono-cytogenes, aerobic gram-negative bacilli	Ampicillin 2 gm IV q4h, plus cefotaxime 2 gm IV q4h, or ceftriaxone 2 gm IV q12h
*Vancomycin 1.0 gm IV q12h should be added to empiric regimens when highly penicillin- or cephalosporin-resistant pneumococcal meningitis is suspected.		

B. If the patient has focal neurologic findings or papilledema, a computed tomographic (CT) scan of the head should be performed before lumbar puncture to rule out the possibility of an intracranial mass lesion; lumbar puncture increases the risk of cerebral herniation in this setting.

C. Emergent empiric antimicrobial therapy should be initiated after blood cultures are obtained and before sending the patient for the CT scan. Antimicrobial therapy should begin within 30 minutes of the patient's presentation to the hospital.

Specific Antimicrobial Therapy for Bacterial Meningitis		
Bacterial pathogen	Standard therapy	Alternative therapies
Streptococcus pneumoniae	Cefotaxime or ceftriaxone and vancomycin	Vancomycin and rifampin
Neisseria meningitidis (meningococcus)	Penicillin G or ampicillin	Cefotaxime or ceftriaxone; chloramphenicol
Haemophilus influenzae Beta-lactamase-negative	Ampicillin	Cefotaxime or ceftriaxone
Beta-lactamase-positive	Cefotaxime or ceftriaxone	Chloramphenicol; aztreonam

Enterobacteriaceae	Cefotaxime or ceftriaxone	Aztreonam; trimethoprim-sulfamethoxazole
Pseudomonas aeruginosa	Ceftazidime and intrathecal gentamicin	Aztreonam and intrathecal gentamicin
Listeria monocytogenes	Ampicillin and gentamicin	Trimethoprim-sulfamethoxazole
Streptococcus agalactiae	Ampicillin or penicillin G	Cefotaxime or ceftriaxone; vancomycin
Staphylococcus aureus Methicillin-sensitive Methicillin-resistant	Oxacillin Vancomycin	Vancomycin
Staphylococcus epidermidis	Vancomycin	

- D. **Duration of Therapy.** Seven days of therapy is usually effective for H. influenzae type b meningitis. Meningococcal meningitis is treated for seven days with intravenous penicillin.
- E. Meningitis secondary to enteric gram-negative bacilli should be treated for three weeks. S. pneumoniae meningitis should be treated for 10 to 14 days. Antimicrobial therapy for meningitis caused by L. monocytogenes, Staphylococcus aureus and S. agalactiae should be extended to 14 to 21 days is recommended.
- F. Adjunctive dexamethasone is not routinely administered for adults with meningitis.
- G. **Reduction of Intracranial Pressure**
  1. Reduction of intracranial pressure is necessary in patients with bacterial meningitis accompanied by an altered level of consciousness, dilated poorly reactive or nonreactive pupils, and/or ocular movement disorders.
  2. Intracranial pressures greater than 260 mm of H20 should be reduced by elevation of the head of the bed to 30 degrees, use of hyperosmolar agents (mannitol, glycerol), and dexamethasone. If these methods fail, high-dose barbiturate therapy (which decreases cerebral metabolic demands and cerebral blood flow) may be used. §

Pneumonia

Community-acquired pneumonia is the leading infectious cause of death and is the sixth leading cause of death overall.

- I. **Clinical Diagnosis**
  - A. **Symptoms** of pneumonia usually include fever, chills, malaise and cough. Patients also may have pleurisy, dyspnea, or hemoptysis. Eighty percent of patients are febrile.
  - B. **Physical exam findings** may include tachypnea, tachycardia, rales, rhonchi, bronchial breath sounds, and dullness to percussion over the involved area of lung.

C. **Chest radiograph** usually shows infiltrates. The chest radiograph may reveal signs of complicated pneumonia, such as multilobar infiltrates, volume loss, or pleural effusion. The chest radiograph may be negative very early in the illness because of dehydration or severe neutropenia.

D. **Further testing** is required if there are severe signs and symptoms (heart rate >140 beats per minute, altered mental status, respiratory rate >30 breaths per minute) or underlying diseases, such as diabetes mellitus or heart disease. Additional tests may include a complete blood count, pulse oximetry or arterial blood gas analysis.

E. Patients with more severe illness, older patients and those with underlying diseases should be considered for hospital admission.

II. Laboratory Evaluation

A. **Sputum for Gram stain and culture** should be obtained in hospitalized patients. In a patient who has had no prior antibiotic therapy, a high-quality specimen (>25 white blood cells and <5 epithelial cells/hpf) may help to direct initial therapy.

B. **Blood cultures** are positive in 11% of cases, and they may identify a specific etiologic agent.

C. **Serologic testing for HIV** is recommended in hospitalized patients between the ages of 15 and 54 years. Serologic testing for *Mycoplasma pneumoniae, Legionella* species, *Chlamydia* species, or fungal pathogens is of limited utility in the initial evaluation. **Urine antigen testing** for legionella is indicated in endemic areas for patients with serious pneumonia.

III. Indications for Hospitalization

A. Age >65years

B. Unstable vital signs (heart rate >140 beats per minute, systolic blood pressure <90 mm Hg, respiratory rate >30 beats per minute)

C. Altered mental status

D. Hypoxemia (PO_2 <60 mm Hg)

E. Severe underlying disease (lung disease, diabetes mellitus, liver disease, heart failure, renal failure)

F. Immune compromise (HIV infection, cancer, corticosteroid use)

G. Complicated pneumonia (extrapulmonary infection, meningitis, cavitation, multilobar involvement, sepsis, abscess, empyema, pleural effusion)

H. Severe electrolyte, hematologic or metabolic abnormality (ie, sodium <130 mEq/L, hematocrit <30%, absolute neutrophil count <1,000/mm^3, serum creatinine > 2.5 mg/dL)

I. Failure to respond to outpatient treatment within 48 to 72 hours.

Pathogens Causing Community-Acquired Pneumonia	
More Common	**Less Common**
Streptococcus pneumoniae Haemophilus influenzae Moraxella catarrhalis Mycoplasma pneumoniae Chlamydia pneumoniae Legionella species Viruses Anaerobes (especially with aspiration)	Staphylococcus aureus Gram-negative bacilli Pneumocystis carinii Mycobacterium tuberculosis

IV. Treatment of Community-Acquired Pneumonia

Recommended Drug Therapy for Patients with Community-Acquired Pneumonia		
Clinical Situation	**Primary Treatment**	**Alternative(s)**
Empiric Inpatient Therapy		
Moderately ill	Second- or third-generation cephalosporin cefuroxime, ceftriaxone [Rocephin], cefotaxime [Claforan]	Beta-lactam/beta-lactamase inhibitor (Ampicillin-sulbactam [Unasyn], Ticarcillin-clavulanate [Timentin]). A macrolide is added if legionella infection is suspected
Critically ill	Erythromycin (±rifampin if *Legionella* organisms documented) plus Third-generation cephalosporin with *anti-Pseudomonas aeruginosa* activity or another antipseudomonal agent (eg, imipenem-cilastatin [Primaxin] or ciprofloxacin [Cipro]) plus Aminoglycoside (pending culture results)	

A. Moderately Ill, Hospitalized Patients

1. In addition to S *pneumoniae* and H *influenzae,* more virulent pathogens, such as S *aureus, Legionella* species, aerobic gram-negative bacilli (including *P aeruginosa,* and anaerobes), should be considered in patients requiring hospitalization.

2. Hospitalized patients should receive an intravenous cephalosporin active against S *pneumoniae* and anaerobes (eg, cefuroxime, ceftriaxone [Rocephin], cefotaxime [Claforan]), or a beta-lactam/beta-lactamase inhibitor.

3. When *P aeruginosa* infection is suspected (recent hospitalization, debilitated patient from a nursing home), only antipseudomonal

cephalosporins with activity against this organism should be used (eg, ceftazidime, cefepime [Maxipime], cefoperazone [Cefobid]) along with an aminoglycoside or a quinolone (ciprofloxacin). Two agents should be used when Pseudomonas aeruginosa is suspected.

4. When legionella is suspected (in endemic areas who have cardiopulmonary disease, immune compromise), a macrolide should be added to the regimen. If legionella pneumonia is confirmed, rifampin (Rifadin) should be added to the macrolide.

B. Critically Ill Patients

1. S pneumoniae and Legionella species are the most commonly isolated pathogens, and aerobic gram-negative bacilli are identified with increasing frequency. M pneumoniae, respiratory viruses, and H influenzae are less commonly identified.

2. Erythromycin should be used along with an antipseudomonal agent (ceftazidime, imipenem-cilastatin [Primaxin], or ciprofloxacin [Cipro]). An aminoglycoside should be added for additional antipseudomonal activity until culture results are known.

Common Antimicrobial Agents for Community-acquired Pneumonia in Adults

Type	Agent	Dosage
Oral therapy		
Macrolides	Erythromycin Clarithromycin (Biaxin) Azithromycin (Zithromax)	500 mg PO qid 500 mg PO bid 500 mg PO on day 1, then 250 mg qd x 4 days
Beta-lactam/beta-lactamase inhibitor	Amoxicillin-clavulanate (Augmentin)	500 mg tid or 875 mg PO bid
Quinolones	Ciprofloxacin (Cipro) Levofloxacin (Levaquin) Ofloxacin (Floxin) Trovafloxacin (Trovan)	500 mg PO bid 500 mg PO qd 400 mg PO bid 200 mg PO qd
Tetracycline	Doxycycline	100 m g PO bid
Sulfonamide	Trimethoprim-sulfamethoxazole	160 mg/800 mg (DS) PO bid
Intravenous Therapy		
Cephalosporins Second-generation Third-generation (anti-Pseudomonas aeruginosa)	Cefuroxime (Kefurox, Zinacef) Ceftizoxime (Cefizox) Ceftazidime (Fortaz)	0.75-1.5 g IV q8h 1-2 g IV q8h 1-2 g IV q8h

Beta-lactam/beta-lactamase inhibitors	Ampicillin-sulbactam (Unasyn)	1.5 g IV q6h
	Ticarcillin-clavulanate (Timentin)	3.1 g IV q6h
Quinolones	Ciprofloxacin (Cipro)	400 mg IV q12h
	Levofloxacin (Levaquin)	500 mg IV q24h
	Ofloxacin (Floxin)	400 mg IV q12h
	Trovafloxacin (Trovan)	200 mg IV q24h

C. Antibiotic Resistance

1. Twenty five percent of S. pneumoniae isolates in some areas of the United States were no longer susceptible to penicillin, and 9% are no longer susceptible to extended-spectrum cephalosporins. Patients with more severe pneumonia or recurrent pneumonia are more likely to harbor resistant S. pneumoniae.

2. Pneumonia caused by penicillin-resistant strains of S. pneumoniae should be treated with high-dose penicillin (penicillin G 2-3 MU IV q4h), or cefotaxime (2 gm IV q8h), or ceftriaxone (2 gm IV q12h), or meropenem (Merrem) (500-1000 mg IV q8h), or vancomycin (Vancocin) (1 gm IV q12h).

3. H. influenzae and Moraxella catarrhalis often produce beta-lactamase enzymes, making these organisms resistant to penicillin and ampicillin. Infection with these pathogens is treated with a second-generation cephalosporin, beta-lactam/beta-lactamase inhibitor combination such as amoxicillin-clavulanate, azithromycin, or trimethoprim-sulfamethoxazole.

V. Clinical Course

A. In about 50% of patients, a specific pathogen will be identified, and empirical therapy can be changed to a more specific antibiotic.

B. In hospitalized patients, intravenous therapy can be changed to oral therapy once the clinical condition has stabilized, and fever and leukocytosis have resolved.

C. Most bacterial infections can be adequately treated with 10-14 days of antibiotic therapy. A shorter treatment course of three to five days is possible with azithromycin because of its long half-life. M pneumoniae and C pneumoniae infections require treatment for up to 14 days. Legionella infections should be treated for a minimum of 14 days; immunocompromised patients require 21 days of therapy. §

Pneumocystis Carinii Pneumonia

Pneumocystis carinii pneumonia (PCP) usually occurs at CD4 counts of less than 200 cells/mm^3. The risk increases as the CD4 cell count declines, with a small proportion of cases occurring at CD4 counts higher then 200, and a greater risk of PCP at CD4 counts below 100. Transmission occurs by the respiratory route.

I. **Diagnosis**
  A. **Symptoms of PCP** include progressive dyspnea, nonproductive cough, fever, night sweats, and fatigue. A productive cough may sometimes be noted.
  B. **Risk Factors for PCP.** CD4 <200/mm^3, oropharyngeal thrush, unexplained fever >2 weeks, prior AIDS defining illness (TB, Kaposi's sarcoma), prior bacterial pneumonia, HIV wasting.
  C. **Physical exam** findings may include cyanosis (39%) and rales (33%).
  D. **Diagnostic Procedures**
    1. **Chest x-ray** usually reveals diffuse, interstitial infiltrates that may progress to a diffuse alveolar process; however, x-ray findings can often be normal or atypical.
    2. **Induced Sputum Stain.** If performed properly, induced sputum examination can diagnose 85-95% of cases of PCP. Fluorescent monoclonal antibody staining is highly specific.
    3. **Bronchoalveolar lavage (BAL)** should be performed in patients in whom the level of suspicion for PCP is high and in whom induced sputum examination is negative.
    4. **Diffusion Capacity for Carbon Monoxide (DL$_{CO}$)** may be useful when PCP is suspected but the chest x-ray is normal or atypical.
    5. **High Resolution CT Scan:** Absence of typical changes (ie, ground glass opacities) on this test may be useful to exclude PCP, but results may be falsely positive.

II. **Treatment of Pneumocystis Carinii Pneumonia**
  A. **Trimethoprim-sulfamethoxazole (TMP-SMX, Bactrim, Septra)**
    1. TMP-SMX is first choice therapy; IV therapy consists of 15-20 mg of trimethoprim component/kg/d in 3-4 divided doses x 21 days (20 mL of IV solution in 250 mL of D5W IVPB q8h) [solution for injection: 80/400 mg/5 mL]
    2. Oral therapy consists of two double strength tabs q8h for 21 days.
  B. **Pentamidine** 4 mg/kg/day IV x 21 days.
  C. **Dapsone/Trimethoprim (DAP/TMP)**
    1. This regimen is the second choice therapy if the patient can not tolerate, or fails to respond to, TMP-SMX. This regimen is appropriate in patients who are not acutely ill and who can tolerate oral drugs.
    2. Dapsone, 100 mg PO qd and trimethoprim, 5 mg/kg PO qid x 21 days
  D. **Clindamycin/Primaquine**
    1. Clindamycin 300-450 mg po q6h plus primaquine 15 mg of base PO qd x 21 days; diarrhea, rash, and liver dysfunction are problems **OR**
    2. Clindamycin 600-900 mg IV q8h plus oral primaquine, 15 mg of base, PO qd.
  E. **Adjunctive corticosteroids** are recommended for patients with a room air A-a gradient >30 or a room air pO$_2$ <70 mm Hg
    1. Prednisone 40 mg po bid x 5 days, then 40 mg qd for 5 days, then 20 mg once daily for 11 days. **OR**

2. Methylprednisolone (Solu-Medrol) 30 mg IV q12h x 5 days, then 30 mg IV qd, then 15 mg IV qd for 11 days.

F. Salvage Therapy
   1. Patients who fail TMP-SMX therapy should be reassessed for other possible diagnoses or coexisting pathogens.
   2. Corticosteroids are added if they are not already being used.
   3. The patient should be switched to pentamidine or trimetrexate. Prior use of DDI, DDC, or prior pancreatitis may contraindicate the use of pentamidine.

III. Prophylaxis Against Pneumocystis Carinii Pneumonia

A. CDC Criteria for Initiating Prophylactic Therapy
   1. CD4 cell count <200 cells/mm^3 (the nadir is the primary determinant)
   2. The percentage of CD4 cells <20% of lymphocytes
   3. A previous episode of PCP has occurred
   4. Constitutional symptoms are present, such as thrush or unexplained fever >37.8 degrees C for 2 or more weeks.

B. Prophylaxis is taken indefinitely, and it is continued even if the CD4 count rises above 200 cells/mm^3 ("restored CD4 count").

C. Trimethoprim-Sulfamethoxazole (TMP-SMX, Bactrim, Septra) is the drug of choice; one double-strength tab daily or 3 times a week. TMP-SMZ is preventative against toxoplasmosis and PCP.
   1. Fever, drug rash and nausea frequently occur 9-12 days after the initiation of, and when symptoms are mild, they usually will pass.
   2. **Sulfa Intolerance.** Patients who have a history of rash after use of TMP-SMX should usually be rechallenged. Desensitization with small doses has also been used.
   3. Toxicities of TMP-SMX include leukopenia, thrombocytopenia, elevated liver enzymes, elevated creatinine, elevated amylase, fever, rash (including rare Stevens-Johnson syndrome), and pruritus. It is usually cross-reactive with dapsone.

D. Dapsone is the second choice agent; 50 mg PO bid or 100 mg PO qd; contraindicated in G6PD deficiency.

E. Aerosolized pentamidine (NebuPent) is a third choice agent; 300-mg (one vial in 6 mL sterile water) once a month via jet nebulizer.

F. Dapsone-pyrimethamine. Fourth choice agent; less effective than TMP-SMX. Dapsone 200 mg plus pyrimethamine 75 mg plus folinic acid 250 mg once weekly.

Antiretroviral Therapy and Opportunistic Infections in AIDS

I. Antiretroviral Therapy

A. A combination of three agents is recommended as initial therapy. The preferred options are 2 nucleosides plus 1 protease inhibitor or 1 non-nucleoside. Alternative options are 2 protease inhibitors plus 1 nucleoside or 1 non-nucleoside. Combinations of 1 nucleoside, 1 non-nucleoside, and 1 protease inhibitor are also effective.

B. Nucleoside Analogs
   1. Zidovudine (Retrovir, AZT) 200 mg PO tid or 300 mg PO bid [cap: 100, 300 mg].

    2. Lamivudine (Epivir) 150 mg PO bid [tab: 150 mg].

    3. Stavudine (Zerit) 40 mg PO bid [cap: 15, 20, 30, 40 mg].

    4. Zalcitabine (Hivid) 0.75 mg PO tid [tab: 0.375, 0.75 mg].

    5. Didanosine (Videx) 200 mg PO bid [chewable tabs: 25, 50, 100, 150 mg]; oral ulcers discourage common usage.

    6. Zidovudine 300 mg/ lamivudine 150 mg (Combivir) 1 tab PO bid.

C. Protease Inhibitors

    1. Indinavir (Crixivan) 800 mg PO tid [cap: 200, 400 mg].

    2. Ritonavir (Norvir) 600 mg PO bid [cap: 100 mg].

    3. Saquinavir (Invirase) 600 mg PO tid [cap: 200 mg].

    4. Nelfinavir (Viracept) 750 mg PO tid [tab: 250 mg]

D. Non-nucleoside analogs

    1. Delavirdine (Rescriptor) 400 mg PO tid [tab: 100 mg]

    2. Nevirapine (Viramune) 200 mg PO bid [tab: 200 mg]

E. Antiretroviral therapy during trimethoprim-sulfamethoxazole therapy may increase the marrow suppressing effects of both drugs.

II. Oral Candidiasis

    A. Fluconazole (Diflucan) Acute: 200 mg PO x 1, then 100 mg qd x 5 days
    OR

    B. Ketoconazole (Nizoral), acute: 400 mg po qd 1-2 weeks or until resolved
    OR

    C. Clotrimazole (Mycelex) troches 10 mg dissolved slowly in mouth 5 times/d.

III. Candida Esophagitis

    A. Fluconazole (Diflucan) 200 mg PO x 1, then 100 mg PO qd until improved.

    B. Ketoconazole (Nizorol) 200 mg po bid.

IV. Primary or Recurrent Mucocutaneous HSV. Acyclovir (Zovirax), 200-400 mg PO 5 times a day for 10 days, or 5 mg/kg IV q8h; OR in cases of acyclovir resistance, foscarnet 40 mg/kg IV q8h for 21 days.

V. Herpes Simplex Encephalitis. Acyclovir 10 mg/kg IV q8h x 10-21 days.

VI. Herpes Varicella Zoster

    A. Acyclovir (Zovirax) 10 mg/kg IV over 60 min q8h **OR**

    B. Valacyclovir (Valtrex) 1000 mg PO tid x 7 days [caplet: 500 mg].

VII. Cytomegalovirus infections

    A. Ganciclovir (Cytovene) 5 mg/kg IV (dilute in 100 mL D5W over 60 min) q12h x 14-21 days (concurrent use with zidovudine increases hematological toxicity).

    B. Suppressive Treatment for CMV: Ganciclovir 5 mg/kg IV qd, or 6 mg/kg IV 5 times/wk, or 1000 mg orally tid with food.

VIII. Toxoplasmosis

    A. Pyrimethamine 200 mg PO loading dose, then 50-75 mg qd plus leucovorin calcium (folinic acid) 10-20 mg po qd for 6-8 weeks for acute therapy **AND**

    B. Sulfadiazine (1.0-1.5 gm PO q6h) or clindamycin 450 mg PO qid/600-900 mg IV q6h.

    C. Suppressive Treatment for Toxoplasmosis

        1. Pyrimethamine 25-50 mg PO qd with or without sulfadiazine 0.5-1.0 Gm PO q6h; and folinic acid 5-10 mg PO qd. **OR**

        2. Pyrimethamine 50 mg PO qd; and clindamycin 300 mg PO q6h; and folinic acid 5-10 mg PO qd.

IX. **Cryptococcus Neoformans Meningitis**. Amphotericin B at 0.7 mg/kg/d IV for 14 days or until clinically stable, followed by fluconazole 400 mg qd to complete 10 weeks of therapy, followed by suppressive therapy with fluconazole (Diflucan) 200 mg PO qd indefinitely.

X. **Active Tuberculosis**
   A. Isoniazid (INH) 300 mg PO qd; and rifampin 600 mg PO qd; and pyrazinamide 15-25 mg/kg PO qd (500 mg PO bid-tid); and ethambutol 15-25 mg/kg PO qd (400 mg PO bid-tid).
   B. All four drugs are continued for 2 months; isoniazid and rifampin (depending on susceptibility testing) are continued for a period of at least 9 months and at least 6 months after the last negative cultures.
   C. Pyridoxine (Vitamin B6) 50 mg PO qd, concurrent with INH.

XI. **Disseminated Mycobacterium Avium Complex (MAC)**
   A. Clarithromycin (Biaxin) 500 mg PO bid; or azithromycin (Zithromax) 500-1000 mg PO qd **AND**
   B. Ethambutol 15-25 mg/kg PO qd (400 mg bid-tid) **AND**
   C. Rifabutin 300 mg/d (two 150 mg tablets qd).
   D. **Prophylaxis for MAC**
      1. Clarithromycin (Biaxin) 500 mg PO bid **OR**
      2. Rifabutin (Mycobutin), 300 mg PO qd or 150 mg PO bid.

XII. **Disseminated Coccidioidomycosis**
   A. Amphotericin B 0.8 mg/kg IV qd **OR**
   B. Fluconazole (Diflucan) 400-800 mg PO or IV qd.

XIII. **Disseminated Histoplasmosis**
   A. Amphotericin B 0.5-0.8 mg/kg IV qd, until total dose 15 mg/kg. **OR**
   B. Itraconazole (Sporanox) 200 mg PO bid.
   C. **Suppressive Treatment for Histoplasmosis:** Itraconazole (Sporanox) 200 mg PO bid.

Sepsis

Sepsis is the most common cause of death in medical and surgical ICUs. Mortality ranges from 20% to 60%.

I. **Pathophysiology**
   A. Sources of bacteremia leading to sepsis include the genitourinary, respiratory and GI tracts, and the skin and soft tissues (including catheter sites). The source of bacteremia is unknown in 30% of patients.
   B. Gram-negative organisms are responsible for 50-80% of all cases of septic shock. Gram-positive organisms cause 6-24% of cases. Parasitic infections, disseminated tuberculosis, and systemic fungal disease are less common causes of sepsis.
   C. Escherichia coli is the most frequently encountered gram-negative organism, followed by Klebsiella pneumoniae, Enterobacter species, Serratia marcescens, Pseudomonas aeruginosa, Proteus mirabilis, Providencia, and Bacteroides species. Sepsis is polymicrobic in 16% of cases.
   D. Gram-positive organisms, including Staphylococcus aureus and Staphylococcus epidermidis, are associated with catheter, line-related, or post-surgical infections.
   E. **Bacteremia** is defined as the presence of viable bacteria in the blood.

F. **Systemic inflammatory response syndrome (SIRS)** is defined as two or more of the following:
1. Temperature >38° C or <36° C
2. Heart rate >90 beats/min
3. Respiratory rate >20 breaths/min
4. White blood cell count >12,000 or <4,000 or >10% bands

G. SIRS is commonly caused by infection, but trauma, burns, and pancreatitis can cause this syndrome.

H. **Sepsis** consists of SIRS plus a documented infection.

I. **Severe sepsis** consists of sepsis plus end-organ dysfunction (eg, hypoxemia, oliguria, altered mentation).

J. **Septic shock** is defined as sepsis with hypotension despite fluid resuscitation.

K. **Sepsis-induced hypotension** is defined as a systolic blood pressure <90 mmHg or a reduction of ≥40 mmHg from baseline in the absence of other causes of hypotension.

L. **Multiple organ dysfunction syndrome (MODS)** is defined as the presence of altered organ function in an acutely ill patient such that homeostasis cannot be maintained without intervention.

II. **Clinical manifestations of sepsis**

A. **Fever** is the most common sign of sepsis, although normal body temperatures and hypothermia are common in the elderly. Other clinical signs of sepsis include tachypnea, altered mentation, oliguria, and tachycardia.

B. **Tachycardia.** In the early stages of sepsis, tachycardia is associated with increased cardiac output, peripheral vasodilation, and a warm, well-perfused appearance. As shock develops, vascular resistance continues to fall, hypotension ensues and cardiac output declines. During the later stages of septic shock, vasoconstriction and cold extremities may occur.

C. **Jaundice** attributable to hepatic dysfunction and GI bleeding may also be caused by sepsis.

D. **Adult respiratory distress syndrome (ARDS).** Sepsis is the most frequent predisposing factor to ARDS. It is characterized by increased pulmonary capillary permeability, resulting in increased extravascular lung water, a widening of the alveolar-arterial O_2 gradient, and hypoxemia (PO_2 <65 mmHg).

III. **Laboratory findings**

A. **Respiratory alkalosis** is usually present in the early stages of sepsis. As shock ensues, metabolic acidosis develop.

B. **Leukocytosis** accompanied by an increased percentage of neutrophils is frequently an early finding in sepsis.

C. **Disseminated intravascular coagulation** is seen in patients with profound sepsis. It is indicated by thrombocytopenia, elevated INR and partial thromboplastin times, decreased fibrinogen levels, and elevated levels of fibrin degradation products.

D. **Renal manifestations** of sepsis range from proteinuria to acute tubular necrosis and renal failure. Shock may cause oliguria and azotemia.

IV. **Hemodynamics**

A. Early septic shock causes a drop in systemic vascular resistance, which may precede decreases in blood pressure. Cardiac output rises in response to the fall in systemic blood pressure, which is often referred to as the "hyperdynamic state" in sepsis. Shock results if the increase in cardiac output is insufficient to maintain blood pressure.

B. Systemic vascular resistance can occasionally rise in the late stages of shock, leading to vasoconstriction.

Laboratory Tests for Serious Infections	

Complete blood count, including leukocyte differential and platelet count
Electrolytes
Arterial blood gases
Blood urea nitrogen and creatinine
Urinalysis
INR, partial thromboplastin time, fibrinogen
Serum lactate
	Cultures with antibiotic sensitivities
	    Blood
	    Urine
	    Sputum
	    Drains
	    Wound
	    Endometrium
	    Amniotic fluid
	Chest X-ray
	Adjunctive imaging studies (eg, computed tomography, magnetic resonance imaging, abdominal ultrasound or X-ray)

V. Clinical management of sepsis
A. Resuscitation

1. Initial resuscitation may require 4 to 6 L of crystalloid. Some anecdotal reports have cited the benefits of albumin solutions in the resuscitation of hypotensive patients.

2. Fluid infusion should be titrated to obtain a pulmonary capillary wedge pressure of 10 to 20 mmHg. Other indices of organ perfusion, such as oxygen delivery, serum lactate levels, arterial blood pressure and urinary output should also guide fluid management.

3. Vasopressor and inotropic therapy is necessary if hypotension persists despite fluid resuscitation. Dopamine is a first-line agent for sepsis-associated hypotension because it has combined dopaminergic, alpha-adrenergic, and beta-adrenergic properties. Initial dose is 10 mcg/kg/min, titrated to a systolic blood pressure of >90 mmHg. At dosages that are higher than 5 mcg/kg/min, dopamine has beta-adrenergic inotropic and alpha-adrenergic vasopressor effects.

4. If hypotension persists despite high dosages of dopamine (20 mcg/kg/min), or if dopamine causes excessive tachycardia, norepinephrine or epinephrine infusions may be used. These agents have alpha-adrenergic and beta-adrenergic effects and cause peripheral vasoconstriction and increased cardiac contractility.

5. Dobutamine can be added to increase cardiac output and oxygen delivery through its beta-adrenergic inotropic effects. This agent is particularly useful in the later stages of septic shock, when cardiac output falls.

Commonly Used Vasoactive and Inotropic Drugs	
Agent	**Dosage**
Dopamine	**Renal Perfusion Dose:** 1-3 mcg/kg/min **Cardiac Inotropic Dose:** 5-10 mcg/kg/min **Vasoconstricting Dose:** 10-20 mcg/kg/min
Dobutamine	**Inotropic:** 5-10 mcg/kg/min **Vasodilator:** 15-20 mcg/kg/min
Norepinephrine	**Vasoconstricting dose:** 2-8 mcg/min
Phenylephrine	**Vasoconstricting dose:** 20-200 mcg/min
Epinephrine	**Vasoconstricting dose:** 1-8 mcg/min

B. **Oxygenation and ventilation**. In the patient with sepsis, oxygen therapy should be started if there is arterial hypoxemia: oxygen saturation <90-92% or pAO_2 <60 mmHg.

C. **Treatment of infection**
   1. An infectious focus should be sought. Inspection and culture of potential sites of infection (including tips of intravascular devices) and drainage of abscesses should be completed.
   2. **Blood cultures.** Two to three sets of blood cultures from separate sites should be drawn.
   3. The choice of antibiotics should be based on the suspected sources of infection, gram-stained smears of clinical specimens, the immune status of the patient, and local patterns of bacterial resistance. Aggressive dosing of antibiotics is recommended.
   4. **Initial treatment of life-threatening sepsis** usually consists of a third-generation cephalosporin (ceftazidime, cefotaxime, ceftizoxime), ticarcillin/clavulanic acid, or imipenem. An aminoglycoside (gentamicin, tobramycin, or amikacin) should also be included.
   5. **Methicillin-resistant staphylococci.** When MRSA is suspected, treatment with vancomycin should be included.
   6. **Intra-abdominal or pelvic infections** are likely to involve anaerobes; therefore, treatment should include either ticarcillin/clavulanic acid, ampicillin/sulbactam, piperacillin/tazobactam, imipenem, cefoxitin or cefotetan. An aminoglycoside should be included. Alternatively, metronidazole with an aminoglycoside and ampicillin may be initiated.
   7. **Biliary tract infections.** When the source of bacteremia is thought to be the biliary tract, cefoperazone, piperacillin plus metronidazole, piperacillin/tazobactam, or ampicillin/sulbactam with an aminoglycoside should be used.
   8. **Dosages of antibiotics used in sepsis**
      a. Cefotaxime (Claforan) 2 gm q4-6h.
      b. Ceftizoxime (Cefizox) 2 gm IV q8h.
      c. Cefoxitin (Mefoxin) 2 gm q6h.
      d. Cefotetan (Cefotan) 2 gm IV q12h.
      e. Ceftazidime (Fortaz) 2 g IV q8h.

    f. Ticarcillin/clavulanate (Timentin) 3.1 gm IV q4-6h (200-300 mg/kg/d).
    g. Ampicillin/sulbactam (Unasyn) 3.0 gm IV q6h.
    h. Piperacillin/tazobactam (Zosyn) 3.375-4.5 gm IV q6h.
    i. Piperacillin, ticarcillin, mezlocillin 3 gm IV q4-6h.
    j. Meropenem (Merrem) 1 gm IV q8h.
    k. Imipenem/ Cilastatin (Primaxin) 0.5-1.0 gm IV q6h.
    l. Gentamicin or tobramycin, 2 mg/kg IV loading dose, then 1.7 mg/kg IV q8h.
    m. Amikacin (Amikin) 7.5 mg/kg IV loading dose; then 5 mg/kg IV q8h.
    n. Vancomycin 1 gm IV q12h.
    o. Metronidazole (Flagyl) 500 mg IV q6-8h.
9. **Antibiotic-resistant gram-negative bacilli**. Imipenem or ciprofloxacin may be used if an antibiotic-resistant gram-negative bacilli is suspected.
10.   **Multiple-antibiotic-resistant enterococci**
    a. An increasing number of enterococcal strains are resistant to ampicillin and gentamicin. The incidence of vancomycin-resistant enterococcus (VRE) is rapidly increasing. Some VRE species may be susceptible to chloramphenicol (0.5-1.0 gm IV q6h) or fluoroquinolones.
    b. Quinupristin/dalfopristin (Synercid) is active against most strains of multiple-drug-resistant Enterococcus. §

Peritonitis

Labs: CBC with differential, SMA 12, albumin, LDH, amylase, lactate. PT/PTT, urine, C&S.
Paracentesis
Tube 1 - Cell count and differential (1-2 mL, EDTA purple top tube)
Tube 2 - Gram ctain of sediment, C&S, AFB, fungal C&S (3-4 mL); inject 10-20 mL into anaerobic and aerobic culture bottle.
Tube 3 - Glucose, protein, albumin, LDH, triglyceride, specific gravity, amylase, (2-3 mL, red top tube).
Syringe - pH (3 mL).
Note:. Serum/fluid albumin gradient should be determined.
Other Tests: Plain film of abdomen. CXR PA & LAT, abdominal ultrasound.
Spontaneous Bacterial Peritonitis (nephrotic or cirrhotic):
Option 1:
   -Ampicillin* 2 gm IV q 4-6h; **AND EITHER**
   Cefotaxime (Claforan) 2 gm IV q4-6h **OR**
   Ceftizoxime (Cefizox) 2 gm IV q8h **OR**
   Gentamicin or Tobramycin 1.5 mg/kg IV, then 1 mg/kg q8h (adjust for renal function). Monitor serum levels.
Option 2:
   -Ticarcillin/clavulanate (Timentin) 3.1 gm IV q6h **OR**
   -Piperacillin/tazobactam (Zosyn) 3.375-4.5 gm IV q6h
Option 3:
   -Imipenem/cilastatin (Primaxin) 0.5-1.0 gm IV q6h.
*Vancomycin 1 gm IV q12h if penicillin allergic.

Secondary Bacterial Peritonitis:
Option 1:
    -Cefotetan (Cefotan) 1-2 gm IV q12h **OR**
    -Cefoxitin (Mefoxin) 1-2 gm IV q6h **OR**
    -Ampicillin 2 gm IV q4-6h **AND**
      Gentamicin or tobramycin (aminoglycosides are not recommended in cirrhotics) 100-120 mg (1.5 mg/kg); then 80 mg IV q8h (5 mg/kg/d) **AND**
    Metronidazole 500 mg IV q6-8h
Option 2:
    -Piperacillin/tazobactam (Zosyn) 3.375-4.5 gm IV q6h with an aminoglycoside as above **OR**
    -Ticarcillin/clavulanate (Timentin) 3.1 gm IV q6h (200-300 mg/kg/d) with aminoglycoside as above.
Option 3:
    -Ampicillin/Sulbactam (Unasyn) 1.5-3.0 gm IV q6h with aminoglycoside as above.
Option 4:
    -Imipenem/cilastatin (Primaxin)1.0 gm IV q6h.

Unexplained Fever in Neutropenic Patients

Between 48-60% of neutropenic patients with absolute neutrophil counts (ANC) <500/mm^3 who become febrile will have an infection, and 16%-20% of patients with an ANC of <100/mm^3 have bacteremia.

I. Pathophysiology
  A. Bacteremia is most frequently caused by aerobic gram-negative bacilli (Escherichia coli. Klebsiella pneumoniae, or Pseudomonas aeruginosa), followed by aerobic gram-positive cocci (coagulase-negative staphylococci, viridans streptococci, or S. aureus).
  B. Fungi are common causes of secondary infections among neutropenic patients who have received courses of broad-spectrum antibiotics; however, these organisms can be the cause of primary infection.
  C. The primary sites of infection include the alimentary tract, where cancer chemotherapy-induced mucosal damage allows invasion of opportunistic organisms. Patients with chronic hereditary neutropenia tend to have upper respiratory tract infections, periodontal infections, and skin infections. Damage to the integument by invasive procedures, such as placement of vascular access devices, may serve as a portal for infection.
  D. A single oral temperature of ≥38.3°C (101°F) in the absence of obvious environmental causes is usually considered fever. A temperature of ≥38.0°C (100.4°F) over at least 1 hour indicates a febrile state.
  E. When the neutrophil count decreases to <1,000 cells/mm^3, increased susceptibility to infection can be expected, with the frequency and severity generally inversely proportional to the neutrophil count.

II. Clinical Evaluation
  A. A search should be undertaken for subtle signs and symptoms of inflammation at the sites most commonly infected. These sites are the periodontium; pharynx; lower esophagus; lung; perineum, including the anus; skin lesions; bone marrow aspiration sites; the eye (funduscopic);

vascular catheter access sites; and tissue around the nails. The day of the onset of fever should be assessed in relation to the first day of the last cycle of chemotherapy.

- **B. Two cultures** of blood for bacteria and fungi should be performed.
- **C. Central venous catheters.** Blood samples for culture are obtained from each lumen as well as from a peripheral vein. Quantitative blood cultures may be helpful for comparing venous catheter and peripheral vein specimens. If a catheter entry site is inflamed or draining, exuding fluid should be examined by gram staining and culture for bacteria and fungi. If such lesions are persistent or chronic, stains and cultures for nontuberculous mycobacteria should be obtained.
- **D. Diarrheal stools** believed to be of infectious etiology should be tested for Clostridium difficile toxin and for bacteria (Salmonella, Shigella, Campylobacter, Aeromonas/Plesiomonas, and Yersinia), viruses (rotavirus or cytomegalovirus), or protozoa (Cryptosporidium species).
- **E. Urine cultures** are indicated if signs or symptoms of urinary tract infection exist, a urinary catheter is in place. or the urinalysis results are abnormal. Pyuria may be absent in the presence of urinary tract infection in neutropenic patients.
- **F. Examination of CSF** may be considered if CNS infection is suspected: however, meningeal inflammation and pleocytosis may be absent in neutropenic patients with meningitis. Cultures and stains of CSF for bacteria and fungi are useful if such infections are suspected.
- **G. Chest radiographs** should be obtained whenever signs or symptoms of respiratory tract abnormality are present.
- **H. Skin lesions,** suspected of being infected, should be aspirated or biopsied for cytology, gram staining, and culture.
- **I. Complete blood counts** and measurement of serum transaminases, sodium, potassium, creatinine, and urea nitrogen are needed for supportive care and to monitor for the possible occurrence of drug toxicity.

III. Initial Antibiotic Therapy

- **A.** All febrile patients with neutrophil counts of <500/mm^3 and those with counts of 500-1,000/mm^3 in whom a further decrease can be anticipated should be treated with intravenous broad-spectrum bactericidal antibiotics in maximal dosages. Afebrile patients who are profoundly neutropenic (neutrophil count <500/mm^3) but who have signs or symptoms compatible with an infection, should receive empirical broad-spectrum antibiotics.
- **B. Vancomycin** 1 gm IV q12h, plus ceftazidime (Ceptaz) 2 gm IV q8h **OR**
- **C. Tobramycin plus piperacillin/tazobactam (Zosyn)** 3.375-4.5 gm IV q6h or ticarcillin/clavulanate (Timentin) 3.1 gm IV q6h **OR**
- **D. Imipenem (Primaxin)** 1.0 gm IV q6h or meropenem (Merrem) 1 gm IV q8h monotherapy. §

References

Preface to the 1997 USPHS/IDSA Guidelines for the Prevention of Opportunistic Infections in Persons Infected with HIV.

1997 Guidelines for the Use of Antimicrobial Agents in Neutropenic Patients with Unexplained Fever. Clinical Infectious Diseases 1997; 25:551-73

Hughes W.T. Opportunistic Infections in AIDS Patients. Opportunistic Infections 95:81-93, 1994

Lane HCLaughon B.E. Falloon J., et. al. Recent Advances in the Management of AIDS-related Opportunistic Infections. Ann. Intern. Med. 120:945-955, 1994.

Tunkel A.R, Wispelway B, Scheld W.N: Bacterial meningitis; Recent advances in pathophysiology and treatment. Ann Int Med 112:610,1990.
Pachon J, et al: Severe community acquired pneumonia. Am Rev Respir Dis 142:36973, 1990

Gastroenterology

Ziad Tannous, MD

Upper Gastrointestinal Bleeding

I. **Clinical evaluation**
   A. Initial evaluation of upper GI bleeding should estimate the duration of hematemesis (vomiting bright red blood or coffee ground material), and volume of bleeding. A history of bleeding occurred after forceful vomiting (Mallory-Weiss Syndrome) should be sought.
   B. Abdominal pain, melena, hematochezia (bright red blood per rectum), history of peptic ulcer, or cirrhosis prior bleeding episodes may be present.
   C. **Precipitating factors.** Use of aspirin, nonsteroidal anti-inflammatory agents, or anticoagulants should be sought.

II. **Physical examination**
   A. **General:** Pallor and shallow rapid respirations may be present; tachycardia indicates a 10% blood volume loss; postural hypotension, with an increase in pulse of 20 and a decrease in systolic of 20, indicates a 20-30% loss.
   B. **Skin:** Delayed capillary refill, stigmata of liver disease (jaundice, spider angiomas, parotid gland hypertrophy) should be sought.
   C. **Chest:** Gynecomastia (cirrhosis).
   D. **Abdomen:** Scars, tenderness, masses, hepatomegaly, dilated abdominal veins should be evaluated. Stool gross or occult blood should be completed.

III. **Laboratory evaluation**
   A. CBC, SMA 12, liver function tests, amylase, INR/PTT, type and cross PRBC, FFP. CBC q6h.
   B. EKG, UA. CXR, upright abdomen (evaluate for free air under the diaphragm).

IV. **Differential diagnosis of upper bleeding:** Peptic ulcer, gastritis, esophageal varices, Mallory Weiss tear (gastroesophageal junction tear caused by vomiting or retching), esophagitis, swallowed blood from epistaxis, malignancy (esophageal, gastric), angiodysplasias, aorto-enteric fistula, hematobilia.

V. **Diagnostic and therapeutic approach to upper gastrointestinal bleeding**
   A. If the bleeding appears to have stopped or has significantly slowed, medical therapy with H2 blockers, and saline lavage is usually all that is required.
   B. A minimum of two 14-16 gauge IV lines should be placed. 1-2 liters of normal saline solution should be infused until blood is ready, then transfuse PRBC's as fast as possible. An estimate of blood transfusion requirement should be based on blood loss rate and vital signs (typically 2-6 units PRBCs are needed). Type O negative blood is given in emergent situations.
   C. A large bore nasogastric tube should be placed, followed by lavage with 2 L of room temperature tap water. The tube should then be connected to low intermittent suction, and the lavage should be then repeated hourly. The NG tube may be removed when bleeding is no longer active.

    D. Oxygen is administered by nasal cannula, guided by pulse oximetry. Urine output should be monitored.

    E. Serial hematocrits should be checked, and maintained greater than 30%. Coagulopathy should be assessed and corrected if necessary with fresh frozen plasma. A pulmonary artery catheterization (Swan-Ganz) should be used to assess the effectiveness of resuscitation in unstable patients.

    F. Definitive diagnosis requires upper endoscopy, at which time electrocoagulation of bleeding sites may be completed.

VI. Mallory-Weiss syndrome

    A. This disorder is defined as a mucosal tear at the gastroesophageal junction, frequently following forceful retching and vomiting.

    B. Treatment is supportive, and the majority of patients stop bleeding spontaneously. Endoscopic coagulation or operative suturing may rarely be necessary.

VII. **Acute medical treatment of peptic ulcer disease**

    A. Ranitidine (Zantac) 50 mg IV bolus, then continuous infusion at 6.25-12.5 mg/h [150-300 mg in 250 mL D5W over 24h (11 cc/h)], or 50 mg IV q6-8h **OR**

    B. Cimetidine (Tagamet) 300 mg IV bolus, then continuous infusion at 37.5-50 mg/h (900 mg in 250 mL D5W over 24h), or 300 mg IV q6-8h **OR**

    C. Famotidine (Pepcid) 20 mg IV q12h. §

Variceal Bleeding

Hemorrhage from esophageal and gastric varices is a severe complication of chronic liver disease.

I. Clinical evaluation

    A. Variceal bleeding should be considered in any patient who presents with significant upper gastrointestinal bleeding. Some patients with liver disease do not exhibit the classic signs of cirrhosis (eg, spider angiomas, palmar erythema, leukonychia, clubbing, parotid enlargement, Dupuytren's contracture).

    B. Jaundice, lower extremity edema and ascites are indicative of decompensated liver disease.

    C. The severity of the bleeding episode can be assessed on the basis of the presence of orthostatic changes (eg, resting tachycardia, postural hypotension), which indicates that about one third or more of blood volume has been lost.

    D. If the patient's sensorium is altered because of hepatic encephalopathy, the risk of aspiration mandates endotracheal intubation.

    E. Placement of a large-caliber nasogastric tube (22 F or 24 F) permits lavage for removal of blood and clots in preparation for endoscopy.

    F. Lavage should be performed with tap water, because saline may contribute to retention of sodium and water.

II. Resuscitation

    A. Blood should be replaced as soon as possible. While blood for transfusion is being made available, intravascular volume should be replenished with intravenous albumin in isotonic saline solution (Albuminar-5) or normal saline solution if the patient does not have ascites or evidence of decompensation.

B. Once euvolemia is established, intravenous infusion should be changed to solutions with a lower sodium content (5% dextrose with ½ or ¼ normal saline).

C. Fresh frozen plasma is administered for patients who have been given massive transfusions; in such cases, calcium should be replaced. FFP is also indicated for patients with coagulopathy.

D. Blood should be transfused to maintain a hematocrit of at least 30%. Serial hematocrit estimations should be obtained during continued bleeding. Values may, however, be inaccurate after acute blood loss.

III. Treatment of variceal hemorrhage

A. Pharmacologic agents

    1. Octreotide (Sandostatin) 50 mcg IV over 5-10 min, followed by 50 mcg/h for 48 hours (1200 mcg in 250 mL D5W); somatostatin analog; beneficial in controlling hemorrhage.

    2. Vasopressin (Pitressin), a posterior pituitary hormone, causes splanchnic arteriolar vasoconstriction and reduction in portal pressure.

        a. Dosage is 20 units IV over 20-30 min, then 0.2-0.4 units/minute (100 U in 250 mL D5W).

        b. Concomitant use of IV nitroglycerin mitigates the vasoconstrictor effects of vasopressin on the myocardial and splanchnic circulations.

    3. Octreotide or vasopressin should be tapered and discontinued over a 24-hour period once hemorrhage has subsided.

B. Additional treatments should be considered if bleeding continues, as indicated by fresh blood aspirate from the nasogastric tube and the need for continued blood transfusion.

C. Tamponade devices

    1. Bleeding from varices may temporarily be reduced with the tamponade balloon tubes. However, the benefit is temporary, and prolonged tamponade causes severe esophageal ulceration and high rebleeding rate.

    2. The Linton-Nachlas tube is recommended; it has a gastric balloon and several ports in the esophageal component. The tube is kept in place for 6 to 12 hours while preparations for endoscopic or radiologic treatment are being made.

D. Endoscopic management of bleeding varices

    1. Endoscopic sclerotherapy involves injection of a sclerosant into varices. The success of the treatment is enhanced by a second sclerotherapy treatment.

    2. Endoscopic variceal ligation involves placement of tiny rubber bands on varices during endoscopy. There are fewer complications with ligation than with sclerotherapy, but both have comparable efficacy.

E. Surgery

    1. Portal-systemic shunt surgery is the most definitive therapy for bleeding varices. The placement of a shunt creates an anastomosis between portal and systemic veins, allowing decompression of the hypertensive portal venous system and almost complete elimination of rebleeding. However, some of the procedures have a 30-40% rate of hepatic encephalopathy, and there is only a slight survival advantage over medical treatment.

    2. Shunts that preserve protal blood flow are preferred, such as the distal splenorenal and the small-diameter portacaval H-graft shunts.

F. **Transjugular intrahepatic portacaval shunt (TIPS)**
   1. Under fluoroscopy, a needle is advanced into the liver through the internal jugular and hepatic veins, and inserted into a large branch of the portal vein. A balloon is then used to enlarge the track to permit the placement of a stent.
   2. Encephalopathy occurs in about 35% of patients and there is a significant risk of shunt thrombosis or stenosis, requiring dilatation or insertion of a new stent.

IV. **Approach to treatment of variceal hemorrhage**
   A. Patients initially should be given octreotide (Sandostatin) or vasopressin infusion plus nitroglycerin while awaiting endoscopic treatment.
   B. If varices are large, endoscopic ligation is preferred; for active bleeding from a spurting varix, sclerotherapy is best.
   C. Failure of endoscopic therapy warrants the use of a portal-systemic shunt. Liver transplantation should be considered in poor-risk patients and when other therapy fails. §

Lower Gastrointestinal Bleeding

The spontaneous remission rate for lower gastrointestinal bleeding, even with massive bleeding, is 80% (the same as for upper gastrointestinal bleeding). No source of bleeding can be identified in 12%, and bleeding is recurrent in 25%. Bleeding has usually ceased by the time the patient presents to the emergency room.

I. **Clinical evaluation**
   A. The severity of blood loss and hemodynamic status should be assessed immediately. Initial management consists of resuscitation with colloidal solutions (hetastarch [Hespan]) or crystalloid solutions (lactated Ringers solution) and blood products if necessary. The source of bleeding should be sought while the patient is being resuscitated.
   B. The duration and quantity of bleeding are assessed; however, the duration of bleeding is often underestimated and the quantity is often overestimated.
   C. Risk factors that may have contributed to the bleeding should be assessed, such as the use of nonsteroidal anti-inflammatory drugs, anticoagulants, history of colonic diverticulosis, renal failure, coagulopathy, colonic polyps or hemorrhoids.
   D. Patients may have a history of hemorrhoids, diverticulosis, inflammatory bowel disease, peptic ulcer, gastritis, cirrhosis, or esophageal varices.
   E. **Hematochezia.** Bright red or maroon blood per rectum suggests a lower GI source; however, 11-20% of patients with an upper GI bleed will have hematochezia as a result of rapid blood loss.
   F. **Melena.** Sticky, black, foul-smelling stools suggest a source proximal to the ligament of Treitz, but it can also result from bleeding in the small intestine or proximal colon.
   G. **Malignancy** may be indicated by a change in stool caliber, anorexia, weight loss and malaise.
   H. **Associated findings**
      1. **Abdominal pain** may result from ischemic bowel, inflammatory bowel disease, or a ruptured aortic aneurysm.

2. **Painless, massive bleeding** suggests vascular bleeding from diverticula, angiodysplasia or hemorrhoids.
3. **Bloody diarrhea** suggests inflammatory bowel disease or an infectious origin.
4. **Bleeding with rectal pain** is seen with anal fissures, hemorrhoids, and rectal ulcers.
5. **Chronic constipation** suggests hemorrhoidal bleeding. New onset constipation or thin stools suggests a left-sided colonic malignancy.
6. **Blood on the toilet paper or dripping** into the toilet water after a bowel movement suggests a perianal source.
7. **Blood coating the outside of stool** suggests a lesion in the anal canal.
8. **Blood streaking or mixed in with the stool** may result from a polyp or malignancy in the descending colon.
9. **Maroon colored stools** often indicate small bowel and proximal colon bleeding.

II. Physical examination

A. **Postural hypotension** suggests a 20% blood volume loss; whereas, overt signs of shock (pallor, hypotension, and tachycardia) indicate a 30-40% blood loss.

B. **The skin** may be cool and pale with delayed capillary refill if bleeding has been significant.

C. **Stigmata of liver disease,** including jaundice, caput medusae, gynecomastia, and palmar erythema, should be sought because these patients frequently have GI bleeding.

III. Differential diagnosis of lower gastrointestinal bleeding

A. Angiodysplasia and diverticular disease of the right colon account for the vast majority of episodes of acute lower gastrointestinal bleeding.

B. Most acute LGI bleeding originates from the colon; however, 15-20% of episodes arise from the small intestine and the upper gastrointestinal tract.

C. **Elderly patients.** Diverticulosis and angiodysplasia are the most common causes of lower GI bleeding.

D. **Younger patients.** Hemorrhoids, anal fissures, and inflammatory bowel disease (IBD) are more common causes.

IV. Diagnosis and management of lower gastrointestinal bleeding

A. Rapid clinical evaluation and resuscitation should precede diagnostic or therapeutic studies. Intravenous fluids (1-2 liters) should be infused over 10-20 minutes to restore intravascular volume, and blood should be transfused if there is rapid ongoing blood loss or if hypotension or tachycardia is present. Coagulopathy is corrected with fresh frozen plasma or platelets.

B. When small amounts of bright red blood are passed per rectum, the lower gastrointestinal tract can be assumed to be the source.

C. In patients with large-volume maroon stools, nasogastric tube aspiration should be performed to exclude massive upper gastrointestinal hemorrhage.

D. If the nasogastric aspirate contains no blood, then anoscopy and sigmoidoscopy should be performed to determine whether a colonic mucosal abnormality (ischemic or infectious colitis) or hemorrhoids might be the cause of bleeding.

   E. If these measures fail to yield a diagnosis, rapid administration of polyethylene glycol-electrolyte solution (CoLyte or GoLYTELY) should be initiated orally or by means of a nasogastric tube; 4 L of the lavage solution is given over a 2- to 3-hour period. This allows for diagnostic and therapeutic colonoscopy and adequately prepares the bowel should emergency operation become necessary.

V. Definitive management of lower gastrointestinal bleeding

A. Colonoscopy

1. Colonoscopy is the procedure of choice for diagnosing colonic causes of gastrointestinal bleeding. It should be performed after adequate preparation of the bowel. If the bowel cannot be adequately prepared because of persistent, acute bleeding, a bleeding scan or angiography is preferable.

2. Endoscopy may be therapeutic for angiodysplastic lesions, polyps, and tumors, which can be effectively coagulated.

3. If colonoscopy fails to reveal a source for the bleeding, the patient should be observed because, in about 80% of cases, bleeding ceases spontaneously.

B. Bleeding scan

1. The technetium-labeled ("tagged") red blood cell bleeding scan can detect bleeding sites when bleeding is intermittent.

2. If the result is positive, the next step is colonoscopy or angiography.

C. Angiography

1. Selective mesenteric angiography detects arterial bleeding that occurs at a rate of 0.5 mL/min or faster. Diverticular bleeding causes pooling of contrast medium within a specific diverticulum (extravasation).

2. Bleeding angiodysplastic lesions appears abnormal vasculature. When active bleeding is seen with diverticular disease or angiodysplasia, selective arterial infusion of vasopressin is effective in arresting hemorrhage in 90%.

D. Surgery

1. If bleeding continues and no source has been found, surgical intervention is warranted.

2. Surgical resection may be indicated for patients with recurrent diverticular bleeding, or for patients who have had persistent bleeding from colonic angiodysplasia and have required blood transfusions.

3. Treatment of lower gastrointestinal bleeding involves resection of the involved segment.

VI. Angiodysplasia

A. Angiodysplastic lesions are small vascular tufts that are formed by capillaries, veins, and venules, appearing as red dots or spider-like lesions 2 to 10 mm in diameter.

B. Angiodysplastic lesions develop secondary to chronic colonic distention, and they have a prevalence rate of 25% in elderly patients.

C. Even though angiodysplasia may be present throughout the entire colon, the most common site of bleeding is the right colon. Most patients with angiodysplasia have recurrent minor bleeding; however, massive bleeding is not uncommon.

VII. Diverticular disease

A. Diverticular disease is the most common cause of acute lower gastrointestinal bleeding.

    B. Sixty to 80% of bleeding diverticula are located in the right colon. Ninety percent of all diverticula are found in the left colon.

    C. Diverticular bleeding tends to be massive, but it stops spontaneously in 80% of patients, and the rate of rebleeding is only 25%.

VIII. Colon polyps and colon cancers

    A. These disorders rarely cause significant acute LGI hemorrhage. Left-sided and rectal neoplasms are more likely to cause gross bleeding than right sided lesions. Right sided lesions are more likely to cause anemia and occult bleeding.

    B. Diagnosis and treatment consists of colonoscopic excision or surgical resection.

IX. Inflammatory bowel disease

    A. Ulcerative colitis can occasionally cause severe GI bleeding associated with abdominal pain and diarrhea.

    B. Colonoscopy and biopsy is diagnostic, and therapy consists of medical treatment of the underlying disease; resection is required occasionally.

X. Ischemic colitis

    A. This disorder is seen in elderly patients with known vascular disease; abdominal pain may be postprandial and associated with bloody diarrhea or rectal bleeding. Severe blood loss is unusual but can occur.

    B. Abdominal films may reveal "thumbprinting", caused by submucosal edema. Colonoscopy reveals a well-demarcated area of hyperemia, edema, and mucosal ulcerations. The splenic flexure and descending colon are the most common sites.

    C. Most episodes resolve spontaneously; however, vascular bypass or resection may occasionally be required.

XI. Hemorrhoids

    A. Hemorrhoids rarely cause massive acute blood loss. In patients with portal hypertension, rectal varices should be sought.

    B. **Diagnosis** is by anoscopy and sigmoidoscopy. Treatment consists of a high fiber diet, stool softeners, and/or hemorrhoidectomy. §

Acute Pancreatitis

I. Diagnosis of acute pancreatitis

    A. Pancreatitis usually presents as abdominal pain associated with elevated pancreatic enzymes. Pain is typically epigastric or in the left upper quadrant, and the pain is described as constant, dull, or boring; radiation of the pain to the mid-back and worsening in the supine position may occur.

    B. Low-grade fever to 101°F is common. Higher temperature may indicate infectious complications. Acute pancreatitis may present with volume depletion, manifesting as hypotension or shock, because of vomiting, hemorrhage, or third spacing of fluid.

    C. Patients may have a distended abdomen, and epigastric tenderness and localized rebound may be elicited.

    D. Bleeding into the pancreatic bed may rarely manifest as ecchymoses of the flanks (Grey Turner's Sign) or as periumbilical bleeding (Cullen's sign).

II. Etiology. Identification of the etiology of an attack of pancreatitis is essential to prevent recurrences.

    A. Alcohol is the most common cause, and pancreatitis typically occurs after consuming 100 mL of alcohol per day for 5-10 years.

    B. Gallstones

        1. Ultrasonography visualizes gallstones in 75% of patients with "idiopathic" acute pancreatitis.

        2. Conditions that predispose to biliary stones. Prolonged fasting (total parenteral nutrition, dieting), pregnancy.

    C. Hypertriglyceridemia >1000 mg/dL may cause pancreatitis; lipid-reducing therapy will prevent recurrences.

    D. Abdominal trauma. Trauma such as an automobile accident can result in acute pancreatitis.

    E. Postoperative. Pancreatitis may occur after upper abdominal, renal, or cardiovascular surgery.

    F. Hypercalcemia. Pancreatitis has been reported with hypercalcemia.

    G. Pregnancy. Pancreatitis is most likely during the third trimester and in the 6 weeks postpartum; it is usually related to alcohol or gallstones.

    H. Anatomic causes. Duodenal diverticula, choledochoceles, pancreatic or ampullary strictures, pancreas divisum, or tumors.

    I. Infections. Viruses, parasites, and bacteria may cause pancreatitis.

    J. Vasculitis. Pancreatitis may be a manifestation of vasculitis.

    K. Drugs. Nonsteroidal anti-inflammatory drugs, erythromycin, thiazides, dideoxyinosine (ddI), pentamidine, sulfonamides, and 5-aminosalicylate.

    L. Other causes. Endoscopic retrograde cholangiopancreatography, hereditary pancreatitis, scorpion stings (Trinidad), organophosphate insecticides.

III. Laboratory evaluation

    A. Elevated amylase is not pathognomonic for pancreatitis. Ruptured ectopic pregnancy, tubo-ovarian abscess, ovarian cysts, duodenal perforation, and mesenteric infarction may result in moderate hyperamylasemia. Clearance of amylase is reduced in renal failure, resulting in up to a threefold elevation.

    B. In acute pancreatitis the amylase elevation is generally more pronounced than in other settings; values are usually at least 3 times normal. Mild hyperamylasemia may be seen in asymptomatic alcoholics and in acute cholecystitis or cholangitis.

    C. An elevated WBC count is common in pancreatitis.

    D. Isoamylase determination. Distinguishes pancreatic amylase from salivary amylase. Elevation of salivary isoamylase occurs with mumps, pneumonia, lung tumors, and breast or prostate cancers.

    E. Macroamylasemia

        1. An elevation of serum amylase may result from low renal excretion of amylase, and is not an unusual finding in the normal population.

        2. Patients with macroamylasemia and pancreatitis may be diagnosed on the basis of an elevated serum lipase.

    F. Lipase is more specific for pancreas than amylase.

IV. Imaging studies

    A. Radiographic studies

        1. Flat and upright films of the abdomen help exclude perforated viscus (free air under diaphragm).

        2. Nonspecific findings of acute pancreatitis: Adynamic ileus or a sentinel loop (localized jejunal ileus). Pancreatic calcifications may be found with chronic pancreatitis.

B. Ultrasonography
1. Useful for evaluation of the biliary tract for gallstones.
2. Acute pancreatitis is indicated by reduced pancreatic echogenicity, enlargement, or ductal dilation. The pancreas cannot be visualized in 40% because of overlying bowel gas.

C. Computed tomography (CT) scanning
1. Contrast-enhanced CT scans have a sensitivity of 90% and a specificity of 100% for the diagnosis of acute pancreatitis.
2. **CT scan** is valuable in detecting pancreatic macrosis and complications.

D. Endoscopic retrograde cholangiopancreatography (ERCP) is not routinely indicated during an attack of acute pancreatitis, but it may be useful in the following situations:
1. Preoperative evaluation of traumatic pancreatitis.
2. Suspected biliary pancreatitis with severe disease that is not improving and may need sphincterotomy and stone extraction.
3. In patients older than 40 years with no identifiable cause, ERCP is indicated once the attack of pancreatitis has subsided to determine the etiology.

V. Assessment of prognosis

A. Ranson's Criteria
1. Used to assess prognosis early in the course of acute pancreatitis.
2. Overall, mortality from acute pancreatitis is approximately 1% in patients with less than 3 signs, 15% with 3 or 4 signs, 40% with 5 or 6 signs, and 100% with 7 or more signs.

Ranson's Criteria for Alcoholic Pancreatitis

At Admission:	During Initial 48 Hours:
1. Age over 55 years	1. Hematocrit drop >10% points
2. WBC >16,000/mm^3	2. BUN rise >5 mg/dL
3. Blood glucose >200 mg/dL (in a nondiabetic)	3. Arterial PO2 <60 mmHg
4. Serum LDH >350 IU/L	4. Base deficit >4 mEq/L
5. AST >250 U/L	5. Serum calcium <8.0 mg/dL
	6. Estimated fluid sequestration >6 L

Ranson's Criteria for Nonalcoholic Pancreatitis

Admission	Initial 48 hours
1. Age over 70 years	1. Hematocrit drop >10% points
2. WBC >18,000/mm^3	2. BUN rise >2 mg/dL
3. Blood glucose >220 mg/dL (in a nondiabetic)	3. Base deficit >5 mEq/L
4. Serum LDH >400 IU/L	4. Serum calcium <8.0 mg/dL
5. AST >250 U/L	5. Estimated fluid sequestration >4 L

VI. Complications of pancreatitis
A. **Pseudocyst** is a pancreatic fluid collection that may regress, or it may progress to a mature pseudocyst.
B. **Necrotizing pancreatitis** occurs after infection of the necrotic pancreatic tissue, often within 6 days after the episode begins.
C. **Shock, adult respiratory distress syndrome** (ARDS), renal failure, and gastrointestinal bleeding are occasional complications.

VII. Medical management of pancreatitis

A. **Supportive medical care for local and systemic complications.** The majority of patients (>80%) have rapid resolution of the inflammatory process and a noncomplicated course.

B. **Replacement of intravascular volume.** Ringer's lactate, normal saline or colloids (albumin) are administer to restore hemodynamic stability and to maintain a urine output of 0.5-1 cc/kg/h. Monitor central venous pressure and replace calcium and magnesium deficits.

C. **Pancreatic rest.** Oral feeding is withheld until nausea, vomiting, and abdominal pain have subsided. Total parenteral nutrition is usually necessary. Fat emulsions are contraindicated if hypertriglyceridemia is present, and should be withheld if serum amylase and lipase increase after its use. After acute symptoms have resolved, feeding may be started, with gradual progression from liquids to a regular diet.

D. **Nasogastric suction** is used if ileus is present.

E. **Antibiotics.** Routine use of antibiotics is not recommended in most cases of acute pancreatitis. In cases of infectious pancreatitis treatment with cefoxitin, cefotetan, ampicillin/sulbactam, or imipenem is appropriate.
1. Cefoxitin 1-2 gm IV q6h.
2. Cefotetan 1-2 gm IV q12h.
3. Ampicillin/sulbactam 1.5-3.0 gm IV q6h.
4. Imipenem/cilastatin (Primaxin) 500 mg IV q6h.

F. **Analgesics.** Meperidine (Demerol) should be used because morphine may cause spasm of the sphincter of Oddi.

G. **Medical management**
1. Somatostatin 250 mcg IV bolus, followed by 100 mcg/h x 48 hours
OR
2. Octreotide (Sandostatin) 100-200 mcg SC three times per day may improve mortality.
3. Insulin may be needed if there is severe hyperglycemia.
4. Alcohol withdrawal prophylaxis may be required with chlordiazepoxide 25-100 mg IV/IM q6h round the clock x 3 days, thiamine 100 mg IM/IV qd x 3d; folic acid 1 mg IM/IV qd x 3d; multivitamin qd.

VIII. Surgical management of pancreatitis

A. **Surgical management** is indicated to exclude other intra-abdominal processes, or if abscess, necrotizing pancreatitis, or large symptomatic pseudocyst.

B. **ERCP** is indicated for patients with severe gallstone pancreatitis who continue to have severe pain at 24-48 h. If stones are demonstrated, a sphincterotomy should be completed.

IX. Pancreatic pseudocyst

A. **Clinical signs** of pseudocyst include continuing abdominal pain, vomiting, nausea, epigastric tenderness, abdominal mass, and hyperamylasemia. CT and ultrasound are diagnostic.

B. **Pseudocyst management**
1. Pseudocysts are managed expectantly for 6-8 weeks until a mature cyst wall develops.
2. Pseudocysts that are less than 5 cm in diameter usually resolve spontaneously.

3. After a mature cyst wall has developed, internal drainage endoscopically should be performed. A malignant pseudocyst should be excluded by biopsy of cyst wall.
4. Percutaneous, CT guided drainage may be considered after thickening of cyst wall has occurred. §

Hepatic Encephalopathy

I. **History and Physical:** Lethargy, confusion, stupor, and coma. Physical exam may reveal hepatosplenomegaly, ascites, jaundice, spider angiomas, gynecomastia, testicular atrophy, and asterixis.
II. **Labs:** Ammonia, CBC, electrolyte panel, liver profile, PT/PTT, ABG, hepatitis panel. UA. CXR, ECG, urine and blood drug screen. Blood and urine cultures.
III. **General Measures:** Avoid sedatives, diuretics, NSAIDs or hepatotoxic drugs. Turn patient q2h while awake, chart stools. Foley to closed drainage.
IV. **Precipitating factors** should be sought, such as infection, portosystemic shunting, hypokalemia and alkalosis, GI bleeding, large protein meal and renal failure.
V. **Treatment**
    A. Lactulose 30-45 mL PO q1h x 3 doses, then 15-45 mL PO bid-qid titrate to produce 2-4 soft stools/d **OR**
    B. Lactulose enema (300 mL of lactulose in 700 mL of tap water) 250 mL PR q6h (clamp rectal tube for 45 min) **OR**
    C. Neomycin, 0.5-1.0 gm PO/NG q4-6h, is given if encephalopathy persists despite lactulose; avoid if azotemic **OR**
    D. Metronidazole 800 mg/d for one week.
VI. **Nutrition and Other Measures**
    A. Protein restriction: 20 gm/d and increase by 10 gm every 3-5 days until protein tolerable is reached.
    B. Increase fiber intake (vegetable).
    C. Ornithine aspirate (ammonia detoxifying agent) 9 gm PO tid.
    D. Zinc supplementation 600 mg/d.

References
Peterson WL; Barnett CC; Smith HJ; et.al: Routine Early Endoscopy in Upper-gastrointestinal-tract Bleeding. N Engl J Med 304:925, 1981.
Keller FS; Rosch J: Value of Angiography in Diagnosis and Therapy of Acute Upper Gastrointestinal Hemorrhage. Dig Dis Sci 26:78s, 1981.
Som P; Oster ZH; Atkins HL; Et.al.: Detection of Gastrointestinal Blood Loss with 99mTc-labeled, Heat-treated Red Blood Cells. Radiology 138:207, 1981.
Dawson J; Cockel R: Ranitidine in Acute Upper Gastrointestinal Hemorrhage. Be Med J 285:476, 1982.
Besson I, et al: Sclerotherapy with or without octreotide for acute variceal bleeding, N Eng J Med 333(9): 555-60, 1995.
Adams L; Soulen MC. TIPS: a New Alternative for the Variceal Bleeder. Am J Crit Care 2:196, 1993.
Grate ND: Diagnosis and treatment of gastrointestinal bleeding secondary to protal hypertension. AJG 1997; 92(7): 1081-91
Riordan SM; Williams R: Treatment of hepatic encephalopathy. NEJM 1997; 337(7): 473-79
Haber PS; Perola EC; Wilson JS: Clinical update: management of acute pancreatitis. J of hepatology 1997; 12(3): 189-97

Toxicology

Kuldip Gill, MD

Poisoning and Drug Overdose

I. **Management of Poisoning and Drug Overdose:**
   A. Stabilize vital signs; maintain airway, breathing and circulation.
   B. Consider intubation if patient has depressed mental status and is at risk for aspiration or respiratory failure.
   C. Establish IV access and administer oxygen.
   D. Draw blood for baseline labs (see below).
   E. If altered mental status is present, administer D50W 50 mL IV push, followed by naloxone (Narcan) 2 mg IV, followed by thiamine 100 mg IV.
   F. If no improvement, evaluate for other causes of altered mental status.

II. **Gastrointestinal Decontamination**
   A. **Gastric Lavage**
      1. **Contraindications:**   Acid, alkali, hydrocarbon, or sharp object ingestion.
      2. Consider intubation for airway protection if depressed mental status.
      3. Place the patient in Trendelenburg's position and left lateral decubitus. Insert a large bore (32-40) french Ewald orogastric tube. A smaller NG tube may be used but may be less effective in retrieving large particles.
      4. After tube placement has been confirmed by auscultation, aspirate stomach contents and lavage with 200 cc aliquots of saline or water until clear (up to 2 L).
      5. Send the first 100 cc for toxicology analysis.
   B. **Activated Charcoal (AC)**
      1. Not effective for alcohols, aliphatic hydrocarbons, caustics, cyanide, elemental metals (boric acid, iron, lithium, lead), or pesticides.
      2. Oral or nasogastric dose is 50 gm mixed with sorbitol. Repeat dose of 25-50 gm q4-6h for 24-48 hours if massive ingestion, sustained release products, tricyclic antidepressants, phenothiazines, sertraline, paroxetine, carbamazepine, digoxin, phenobarbital, phenytoin, valproate, salicylate, doxepin, or theophylline were ingested.
      3. Give oral cathartic with charcoal (70% sorbitol). Use magnesium with caution in renal insufficiency.
   C. **Whole Bowel Irrigation (WBI)**
      1. Can prevent further absorption in cases of massive ingestion, delayed presentation, or in overdoses of enteric coated or sustained release pills.
      2. May be useful in eliminating objects, such as batteries, or ingested packets of drugs.
      3. Administer GoLytely, or Colyte orally at 1.6 - 2.0 l/hour until fecal effluent is clear. Contraindicated in patients with ileus.
   D. **Hemodialysis:** Indications include ingestion of phenobarbital, theophylline, chloral hydrate, salicylate, ethanol, lithium, ethylene glycol, isopropyl alcohol, procainamide, and methanol, or severe metabolic acidosis.

E. Hemoperfusion (charcoal or resin):
1. May be more effective than hemodialysis **except** for bromides, heavy metals, lithium, and ethylene glycol.
2. Effective for disopyramide, phenytoin, barbiturates, theophylline.

Toxicologic Syndromes

I. Characteristics of Common Toxicologic Syndromes:
A. **Cholinergic Poisoning:** Salivation, bradycardia, defecation, lacrimation, emesis, urination, miosis.
B. **Anticholinergic Poisoning:** Dry skin, flushing, fever, urinary retention, mydriasis, thirst, delirium, conduction delays, tachycardia, ileus.
C. **Sympathomimetic Poisoning:** Agitation, hypertension, seizure, tachycardia, mydriasis, vasoconstriction.
D. **Narcotic Poisoning:** Lethargy, hypotension, hypoventilation, miosis, coma, ileus.
E. **Withdrawal Syndrome:** Diarrhea, lacrimation, mydriasis, cramps, tachycardia, hallucination.
F. **Common Causes of Toxic Seizures:** Amoxapine, anticholinergics, camphor, carbon monoxide, cocaine, ergotamine, isoniazid, lead, lindane, lithium, LSD, parathion, phencyclidine, phenothiazines, propoxyphene propranolol, strychnine, theophylline, tricyclic antidepressants, normeperidine (metabolite of meperidine), thiocyanate.
G. **Common Causes of Toxic Cardiac Arrhythmias:** Arsenic, beta-blockers, chloral hydrate, chloroquine, clonidine, calcium channel blockers, cocaine, cyanide, carbon monoxide, digitalis, ethanol, phenol, phenothiazine, tricyclics.
H. **Salicylate poisoning:** Fever, respiratory alkalosis, or mixed acid-base disturbance, hyperpnea, hypokalemia, tinnitus.
I. **Extrapyramidal syndromes:** Dysphagia, dysphonia, trismus, rigidity, torticollis, laryngospasm.

Acetaminophen Overdose

I. Clinical Features
A. Acute lethal dose = 13 - 25 g. Acetaminophen is partly metabolized to N-acetyl-p-benzoquinonimine which is conjugated by glutathione. Hepatic glutathione stores can be depleted in acetaminophen overdose, leading to centrilobular necrosis.
B. Signs and Symptoms
1. Liver failure occurs 3 days after ingestion if untreated. Liver failure presents with right upper quadrant pain, elevated liver function tests, coagulopathy, hypoglycemia, renal failure and encephalopathy.
II. Treatment
A. **Gastrointestinal Decontamination:** Gastric lavage followed by activated charcoal. Remove residual charcoal with saline lavage prior to giving N-Acetyl-Cysteine (NAC).
B. Check acetaminophen level 4 hours post ingestion. Use nomogram to determine if treatment is necessary (see next page). Start treatment if

level is above the nontoxic range or if the level is potentially toxic but the time of ingestion is unknown.

C. Therapy must start no later than 8-12 hours after ingestion. Treatment after 16-24 hours of non-sustained release formulation is significantly less effective, but should still be accomplished.

D. Oral N-Acetyl-Cysteine (Mucomyst): 140 mg/kg PO followed by 70 mg/kg PO q4h x 17 doses (total 1330 mg/kg over 72 h). Repeat loading dose if emesis occurs.

E. If oral route is not possible, the following protocol is available (but not FDA approved): NAC 150 mg/kg in 200 mL D5W IV over 15 min, followed by 50 mg/kg in 500 mL D5W IV over 4h, followed by 100 mg/kg in 1000 mL D5W IV over next 16 hours. Filter solution through 0.22 micron filter prior to administration. Complete all PO/NG/IV doses even after acetaminophen level falls below critical value.

F. Hemodialysis and hemoperfusion are somewhat effective, but should not take the place of NAC treatment.

Cocaine Overdose

I. **Clinical Evaluation**
   A. Cocaine can be used intravenously, smoked, ingested, or inhaled nasally. The effect of oral cocaine is equivalent to the intranasal route.
   B. Street cocaine comes in unreliable concentrations, and often is cut with other substances including amphetamines, LSD, PCP, heroin, strychnine, lidocaine, talc, and quinine.
   C. One-third of fatalities occur within 1 hour, with another third occurring 6 to 24 h later.
   D. Be aware of "body packers" who transport cocaine by swallowing well wrapped packets, and "body stuffers" who hastily swallow packets of cocaine to avoid arrest.

II. **Clinical Features**
   A. **CNS:** Sympathetic stimulation, agitation, seizures, tremor, headache, subarachnoid hemorrhage, ischemic cerebral stoke, psychosis, hallucinations, fever, mydriasis, formication (sensation of insects crawling on skin).
   B. **Cardiovascular:** Atrial and ventricular arrhythmias, myocardial infarction, hypertension, hypotension, myocarditis, aortic rupture, cardiomyopathy.
   C. **Pulmonary:** Noncardiogenic pulmonary edema, pneumomediastinum, alveolar hemorrhage, hypersensitivity pneumonitis, bronchiolitis obliterans.
   D. **Other:** Rhabdomyolysis, mesenteric ischemia, hepatitis.

III. **Treatment:**
   A. Supportive care is administered because no antidote exists.
   B. GI Decontamination, including repeated activated charcoal, whole bowel irrigation and endoscopic evaluation is provided if oral or packet ingestion is suspected.
   C. Treat hyperadrenergic symptoms with benzodiazepines such as diazepam.
   D. **Seizures**
      1. Treat with diazepam, phenytoin, or phenobarbital.

    2. Evaluate for other possible causes of seizures such as subarachnoid hemorrhage, hypoxemia, and hypoglycemia.

E. Arrhythmias

1. Treat hyperadrenergic state and supraventricular tachycardia with diazepam and propranolol.
2. Treat ventricular arrhythmias with lidocaine or propranolol may be required.

F. Hypertension

1. Use diazepam first for tachycardia and hypertension.
2. If no response, use labetalol for alpha and beta blocking effects.
3. If hypertension remains severe, consider sodium nitroprusside and esmolol drips.

G. Myocardial Ischemia and Infarction

1. Treat with thrombolysis, heparin, aspirin, beta-blockers, nitroglycerin.
2. Control hypertension and consider possibility of CNS bleeding before using thrombolytic therapy. May use calcium channel blockers for coronary spasm if not contraindicated.

Cyclic Antidepressant Overdose

I. Clinical Features

A. Cyclic antidepressants have a large volume of distribution (15-40 L/kg), high lipid solubility, high protein binding. Antidepressants have prolonged body clearance rates, and can not be removal by forced diuresis, hemodialysis, and hemoperfusion.

B. Delayed absorption is common because of decreased GI motility from anticholinergic effects.

C. Cyclic antidepressants undergo extensive enterohepatic recirculation.

D. **CNS:** Lethargy, coma, hallucinations, seizures, myoclonic jerks.

E. **Anticholinergic crises:** Blurred vision, dilated pupils, urinary retention, dry mouth, ileus, hyperthermia.

F. **Cardiac:** Hypotension, ventricular tachyarrhythmias, sinus tachycardia.

G. **EKG:** Sinus tachycardia, right bundle branch block, right axis deviation, increased PR and QT interval, QRS >100 msec, or right axis deviation. Prolongation of the QRS width is a more reliable predictor of CNS and cardiac toxicity than the TCA level.

II. Treatment

A. Gastrointestinal Decontamination and Systemic Drug Removal

1. Magnesium citrate 300 mL via nasogastric tube x 1 dose.
2. Activated charcoal premixed with sorbitol 50 gm via nasogastric tube q4-6h around-the-clock until TCA level decreases to therapeutic range. Maintain the head-of-bed at a 30-45 degree angle to prevent aspiration.

3. **Cardiac Toxicity**

    a. Alkalinization is a cardioprotective measure and it has no influence on drug elimination. Treatment goal is to achieve an arterial pH of 7.50-7.55.

    b. If mechanical ventilation is necessary, hyperventilate to maintain desired pH.

    c. Administer sodium bicarbonate 50-100 mEq (1-2 amps or 1-2 mEq/kg) IV over 5-10 min. Followed by infusion of sodium bicarbonate, 2 amps in 1 liter of D5W at 100-150 cc/h. Adjust IV rate to maintain desired pH.

4. Seizures
   a. Lorazepam or diazepam IV followed by phenytoin.
   b. Physostigmine, 1-2 mg slow IV over 3-4 min, is necessary if seizures continue.

Digoxin Overdose

I. Clinical Features
   A. Therapeutic window is 0.8-2.0 ng/mL.
   B. Drug-drug interactions that increase digoxin levels include verapamil, quinidine, amiodarone, flecainide, erythromycin, and tetracycline.
   C. Hypokalemia, hypomagnesemia and hypercalcemia enhance digoxin toxicity.
   D. CNS: Confusion, lethargy; yellow-green visual halo.
   E. Cardiac: Most common dysrhythmias include ventricular tachycardia or fibrillation; variable atrioventricular block, atrioventricular dissociation; sinus bradycardia, junctional tachycardia, premature ventricular contractions.
   F. GI: Nausea, vomiting.
   G. Metabolic: Hypokalemia enhances the toxic effects of digoxin on the myocardial tissue and may be present in patients on diuretics.

II. Treatment
   A. Gastrointestinal Decontamination: Gastric lavage, followed by repeated doses of activated charcoal is effective; hemodialysis is ineffective.
   B. Treat bradycardia with atropine, isoproterenol, and cardiac pacing.
   C. Treat ventricular arrhythmias with lidocaine or phenytoin. Avoid procainamide and quinidine as they may be proarrhythmic and slow AV conduction.
   D. Electrical DC cardioversion may be dangerous in severe toxicity.
   E. Hypomagnesemia and hypokalemia should be corrected.
   F. Digibind (Digoxin - specific Fab antibody fragment):
      1. Indication: life threatening arrhythmias refractory to conventional therapy.
      2. Dosage of Digoxin immune Fab:

$$\text{(number of 40 mg vials)} = \frac{\text{Digoxin level (ng/mL) x body weight (kg)}}{100}$$

   3. Dissolve the digoxin immune Fab in 100-150 mL of NS and infuse IV over 15-30 minutes. Use a 0.22 micron in-line filter during infusion.
   4. Hypokalemia, heart failure, and anaphylaxis may occur. The complex is renally excreted; after administration, serum digoxin levels may be high and inaccurate because both free and bound digoxin is measured.

Ethylene Glycol Ingestion

I. **Clinical Features**
   A. **Ethylene glycol** is found in antifreeze, detergents, and polishes.
   B. **Toxicity:** Half-life 3-5 hours; the half-life increases to 17 hours if coingested with alcohol; minimal lethal dose 1.0-1.5 cc/kg; lethal blood level 200 mg/dL.
   C. Anion gap metabolic acidosis and severe osmolar gap is often present.
   D. CNS depression; cranial nerve dysfunction (facial and vestibulocochlear palsies).
   E. GI symptoms such as flank pain; oxalate crystals in urine sediment; hypocalcemia (due to calcium oxalate formation); tetany, seizures, and prolonged QT may occur.

II. **Treatment**
   A. Fomepizole (Antizol) loading dose 15 mg/kg IV; then 10 mg/kg IV q12h x 4, then 15 mg/kg IV q12h until ethylene glycol level <20 mg/dL.
   B. Pyridoxine 100 mg IV qid x 2 days and thiamine 100 mg IV qid x 2 days; may increase metabolism of glyoxylate.
   C. If definitive therapy is not immediately available, 3-4 ounces of whiskey (or equivalent) may be given orally.
   D. **Hemodialysis Indications:** Severe refractory metabolic acidosis, crystalluria, serum ethylene glycol level >50 mg/dL; keep glycol level <10 mg/dL.

Isopropyl Alcohol Ingestion

I. **Clinical Features**
   A. **Isopropyl alcohol** is found in rubbing alcohol, solvents, and antifreeze.
   B. **Toxicity:** Lethal dose: 3-4 g/kg
      1. Lethal blood level: 400 mg/dL
      2. Half life = 3 hours
   C. **Metabolism:** Isopropyl alcohol is metabolized to acetone.
   D. Toxicity is characterized by an anion gap metabolic acidosis with high serum ketone level; mild osmolar gap; mildly elevated glucose.
   E. CNS depression, headache, nystagmus; cardiovascular depression, abdominal pain and vomiting, and pulmonary edema.

II. **Treatment**
   A. Provide supportive care. No antidote is available; ethanol is not indicated.
   B. **Hemodialysis:** Indications: refractory hypotension, coma, potentially lethal blood levels.

Methanol Ingestion

I. Clinical Features

A. **Methanol** is found in antifreeze, Sterno, cleaners, and paints.

B. **Toxicity:**
1. 10 cc causes blindness
2. Minimal lethal dose = 1-5 g/kg
3. Lethal blood level = 80 mg/dL
4. Symptomatic in 40 minutes to 72 hours.

C. **Signs and Symptoms:**
1. Severe osmolar and anion gap metabolic acidosis.
2. Visual changes occur because of optic nerve toxicity, leading to blindness.
3. Nausea, vomiting, abdominal pain, pancreatitis, and altered mental status.

II. Treatment

A. Ethanol 10% is infuse in D5W as 7.5 cc/kg load then 1.4 cc/kg/h drip to keep blood alcohol level between 100-150 mg/dL. Continue therapy until methanol level is below 20-25 mg/dL.

B. Give folate 50 mg IV q4h to enhance formic acid metabolism.

C. Correct acidosis and electrolyte imbalances.

D. **Hemodialysis:** Indications: peak methanol level >50 mg/dL; formic acid level >20 mg/dL; severe metabolic acidosis; acute renal failure; any visual compromise.

Iron Overdose

I. Clinical Features

A. Toxicity is caused by free radical organ damage and damage to the GI mucosa, liver, kidney, heart, and lungs. The cause of death is usually shock and liver failure.

Toxic dosages and serum levels	
Nontoxic	<10-20 mg/kg (0-100 mcg/dL)
Toxic	>20 mg/kg (350-1000 mcg/dL)
Lethal	>180-300 mg/kg (>1000 mcg/dL)

B. **Two Hours After Ingestion:** Severe hemorrhagic gastritis; vomiting, diarrhea, lethargy, tachycardia, and hypotension.

C. **Twelve Hours After Ingestion:** Improvement and stabilization.

D. **12-48 Hours After Ingestion:** GI bleeding, coma, seizures, pulmonary edema, circulatory collapse, hepatic and renal failure, coagulopathy, hypoglycemia, and severe metabolic acidosis.

II. Treatment

A. Administer deferoxamine if iron levels reach toxic values. Deferoxamine 100 mg binds 9 mg of free elemental iron.

    B. Deferoxamine Dosage: 10-15 mg/kg/hr IV infusion.
    C. Treat until 24 hours after vin rose colored urine clears. Serum iron levels during chelation are not accurate.
    D. Deferoxamine can cause hypotension, allergic reactions such as pruritus, urticarial wheals, rash, anaphylaxis, tachycardia, fever, and leg cramp.
    E. Gastrointestinal Decontamination
        1. Charcoal is not effective in absorbing elemental iron. Evaluate x-rays for remaining iron tablets. Consider whole bowel lavage if iron pills are past the stomach and cannot be removed by gastric lavage (see page 93).
        2. Hemodialysis is considered for severe toxicity.

Lithium Overdose

I. Clinical Features
    A. Lithium has a narrow therapeutic window of 0.8-1.2 mEq/l.
    B. Drug-drug interactions will increase lithium levels: NSAIDs, phenothiazines, thiazide and loop diuretics (by causing hyponatremia).
    C. Toxicity:
        1.5-3.0 mEq/l = moderate toxicity
        3.0-4.0 mEq/l = severe toxicity
    D. Toxicity in chronic lithium users occurs at much lower serum levels than with acute ingestions.
    E. Common manifestations include seizures, encephalopathy, hyperreflexia, tremor, nausea, vomiting, diarrhea, hypotension; nephrogenic diabetes insipidus, hypothyroidism.
    F. Conduction block and dysrhythmias are rare, but reversible T wave depression may occur.

II. Treatment
    A. Correct hyponatremia with aggressive normal saline hydration.
    B. Follow lithium levels until <1.0 mEq/l and watch for rebound as levels may increase from intracellular stores.
    C. Forced Solute Diuresis: Hydrate with normal saline infusion to maintain urine output at 2-4 cc/kg/hr; use furosemide (Lasix) 40-80 mg IV doses as needed.
    D. GI Decontamination
        1. Administer gastric lavage. Activated charcoal is ineffective. Whole bowel irrigation may be useful.
        2. Indications for Hemodialysis: Level >4 mEq/l; chronic ingestion with symptoms; CNS or cardiovascular impairment with level of 2.5-4.0 mEq/l.

Salicylate Overdose

I. **Clinical Features**
   A. **Toxicity**
      150-300 mg/kg - mild toxicity
      300-500 mg/kg - moderate toxicity
      >500 mg/kg - severe toxicity
   B. Chronic use can cause toxicity at much lower levels (ie, 25 mg/dL) than occurs with acute use.
   C. **Acid/Base Abnormalities:** Patients present initially with a respiratory alkalosis because of central hyperventilation; later an anion gap metabolic acidosis occurs.
   D. **CNS:** Tinnitus, lethargy, irritability, seizures, coma, cerebral edema.
   E. **GI:** Nausea, vomiting, liver failure, GI bleeding.
   F. **Cardiac:** Hypotension, sinus tachycardia, AV block, wide complex tachycardia.
   G. **Pulmonary:** Non-cardiogenic pulmonary edema, adult respiratory distress syndrome.
   H. **Metabolic:** Renal failure; coagulopathy because of decreased factor VII; hyperthermia because of uncoupled oxidative phosphorylation. Hypoglycemia may occur in children, but it is rare in adults.

II. **Treatment**
   A. Provide supportive care and GI decontamination. Aspirin may form concretions or drug bezoars, and ingestion of enteric coated preparations may lead to delayed toxicity.
   B. Multiple dose activated charcoal, whole bowel irrigation, and serial salicylate levels are indicated.
   C. Treat hypotension and dehydration vigorously with fluids, and correct electrolytes, especially potassium. Maintain urine output at 200 cc/h or more.
   D. Correct metabolic acidosis with bicarbonate 50-100 mEq (1-2 amps) IVP.
   E. Renal clearance is increased by alkalinization of urine with an IV bicarbonate infusion (2-3 amps in 1 liter of D5W at 150-200 mL/h), keeping the urine pH at 7.5-8.5.
   F. **Hemodialysis or charcoal hemoperfusion**
      1. Indications: Seizures, cardiac or renal failure, intractable acidosis, acute salicylate level >120 mg/dL or chronic level >50 mg/dL (therapeutic level 15-25 mg/dL).
      2. Hemoperfusion is effective in clearance of salicylate, but less effective at correcting electrolyte and acid-base imbalances.

Theophylline Toxicity

I. Clinical Features

A. Drug interactions can increase serum theophylline level, including quinolone and macrolide antibiotics, propranolol, cimetidine, and oral contraceptives.

B. Liver disease or heart failure will decrease clearance.

C. Serum Toxicity levels:
20-40 mg/dL - mild
40-70 mg/dL - moderate
>70 mg/dL - life threatening

D. Toxicity in chronic users occurs at lower serum levels than with short-term users. Seizures and arrhythmias can occur at therapeutic or minimally supra-therapeutic levels.

E. CNS: Hyperventilation, agitation, and tonic-clonic seizures.

F. Cardiac: Sinus tachycardia, multi-focal atrial tachycardia, supraventricular tachycardia, ventricular tachycardia and fibrillation, premature ventricular contractions, hypotension or hypertension.

G. GI: Vomiting, diarrhea, hematemesis.

H. Musculoskeletal: Tremor, myoclonic jerks

I. Metabolic: Decreased potassium, magnesium, phosphate, and increased glucose and calcium.

II. Treatment

A. Gastrointestinal Decontamination and Systemic Drug Removal

1. Activated charcoal premixed with sorbitol, 50 gm PO or via nasogastric tube q4h around-the-clock until theophylline level <20 mcg/mL. Maintain head-of-bed at 30 degrees to prevent charcoal aspiration. Activated charcoal increases theophylline clearance by twofold.

2. Hemodialysis is as effective as repeated oral doses of activated charcoal and should be used when charcoal hemoperfusion is not feasible.

3. **Indications for Charcoal Hemoperfusion:** Coma, seizures, hemodynamic instability, theophylline level >60 mcg/mL; rebound in serum levels may occur after discontinuation of hemoperfusion. Charcoal hemoperfusion increases theophylline clearance by sixfold.

4. **Seizures** are generally refractory to anticonvulsants. High doses of lorazepam, diazepam or phenobarbital should be used; phenytoin is less effective.

5. **Treatment of Hypotension**
   a. Normal saline fluid bolus.
   b. Norepinephrine 8-12 mcg/min IV infusion or
   c. Phenylephrine 0.04-1.8 mg/min IV infusion.

6. **Treatment of Arrhythmias**
   a. Bretylium 5-10 mg/kg bolus, then 2 mg/min IV infusion. Lidocaine should usually be avoided because it has epileptogenic properties.
   b. Esmolol (Brevibloc) 500 mcg/kg/min loading dose, then 50-300 mcg/kg/min continuous IV drip.

Warfarin (Coumadin) Overdose

I. Clinical Management

A. Elimination Measures: Gastric lavage and activated charcoal if recent oral ingestion of warfarin (Coumadin).

B. Reversal of Coumadin Anticoagulation: Coagulopathy may be corrected rapidly or slowly depending on the following factors: 1) Intensity of hypocoagulability, 2) severity or risk of bleeding, 3) need for reinstitution of anticoagulation.

C. Emergent Reversal:

1. Fresh frozen plasma: Replace Vitamin K dependent factors with FFP 2-4 units; repeat in 4 hours if prothrombin time remains prolonged.
2. Vitamin K 25 mg in 50 cc NS to infuse no faster than 1 mg/min; risk of anaphylactoid reactions and shock; slow infusion minimizes risk.

D. Reversal over 24-48 Hours: Vitamin K 10-25 mg subcutaneously. Full reversal of anticoagulation will result in resistance to further Coumadin therapy for several days.

E. Partial Correction: Lower doses of Vitamin K (0.5-1.0 mg) will lower prothrombin time without interfering with reinitiation of Coumadin.

References

The American Academy of Clinical Toxicology and the European Association of Poison Control Centers and Clinical Toxicologists position statement on gut decontamination in acute poisoning. J Toxicol-Clin Toxicol 1997; 35:695-762.

Kelly RA, Smith TW: Recognition and management of digitalis toxicity. The American Journal of Cardiology,69:108G, 1992

Markenson D, Greenberg MD: Cyclic Antidepressant overdose: mechanism to management. Emergency Medicine, 25:49, 1993.

Prescott LF: Treatment of severe acetaminophen poisoning with intravenous acetylcysteine. Arch Intern Med. 1981; 141:386-9

Smilkstein MJ, Bronstein AC, et al.: Acetaminophen overdose: a 48-hour intravenous N-acetylcysteine treatment protocol. Annals of Emergency Medicine, 20:1058, 1991.

Spiller HA, Kreuzelok EP, Grand GA, et al.: A prospective evaluation of the effect of activated charcoal before oral n-acetylcysteine in acetaminophen overdose. Annals of Emergency Medicine, 23:519-523, 1994.

Cooling DS. Theophylline toxicity. Journal of Emergency Medicine, 11 (4):415-25, 1993.

Neurologic Disorders

Ziad Tannous, MD

Ischemic Stroke

Ischemic stroke is the third leading cause of death in the United States and the most common cause of neurologic disability in adults. Rapid evaluation of the stroke patient is essential. The time from stroke to treatment (with t-PA) should be 3 hours or less.

I. **Clinical Evaluation of the Stroke Patient**
   A. A rapid evaluation should determine the time when symptoms started. In patients whose symptoms were present upon awakening, their time of symptom onset is estimated from the last time that the patient's neurological status was known to be normal, or the time just prior to going to sleep. Other diseases that may mimic a stroke, including seizure disorder, hypoglycemia, complex migraine, dysrhythmia or syncope, should be excluded.
   B. Markers of vascular disease such as diabetes, angina pectoris, and intermittent claudication are suggestive of ischemic stroke. A history of atrial fibrillation or MI suggests a cardiac embolic stroke.

II. **Physical Examination**
   A. Assessment should determine whether the patient's condition is acutely deteriorating or relatively stable. Airway and circulatory stabilization take precedence over diagnostic and therapeutic interventions.
   B. **Neurologic Exam.** Evaluation should include the level of consciousness, orientation; ability to speak and understand language; cranial nerve function, especially eye movements and pupil reflexes and facial paresis; neglect, gaze preference, arm and leg strength, sensation, and walking ability.
   C. A semiconscious or unconscious patient probably has a hemorrhage. A patient with an ischemic stroke may be drowsy but is unlikely to lose consciousness unless the infarcted area is large.

III. **CT Scanning and Diagnostic Studies**
   A. All patients with signs of stroke should undergo a noncontrast head CT to screen for bleeding and to rule out expanding lesions such as subdural hematomas, epidural hematomas, or other indications for emergent surgery.
   B. A complete blood count (CBC) including platelets, international normalized ratio (INR), activated partial thromboplastin time (aPTT), serum electrolytes, and a rapid blood glucose should be obtained. ECG, and chest x-ray should be ordered. If the patient is a candidate for thrombolytic therapy, typed and cross-match should be obtained. Arterial blood gas and lumbar puncture should be obtained when indicated.

IV. **Management of Ischemic Stroke**
   A. Labored or weak respirations are an indication for intubation and ventilation. Thrombolytic therapy inclusion and exclusion criteria should be reviewed. Successful treatment of patients with ischemic stroke depends on the ability to treat within three hours of onset, because tissue plasminogen activator has not yet been proved effective beyond this time frame.

Inclusion and Exclusion Criteria for Administration of t-PA

Inclusion Criteria
- Ischemic stroke
- t-PA can be administered within 3 hours of symptom onset
- Measurable neurological deficit
- Clearly defined time of symptom onset

Exclusion Criteria
- Evidence of acute intracerebral or intracranial hemorrhage on non-contrast CT of the head
- Prior stroke, serious head trauma, or intracranial surgery in past three months
- Intracranial neoplasm, arteriovenous malformation, or aneurysm
- Uncontrolled hypertension (ie, blood pressure not reduced to 185/110 or lower within 30 minutes by oral agents, labetalol, or esmolol)
- Rapidly improving or minor neurological symptoms
- Symptoms suggesting subarachnoid hemorrhage
- History of intracranial hemorrhage
- Major surgery in past 14 days
- Known bleeding diathesis
- Gastrointestinal or genitourinary tract bleeding in the past 3 weeks
- Arterial puncture at a non-compressible site in the past 7 days
- Seizure at the onset of stroke
- Prothrombin (PT) time greater than 15 seconds
- Patients on warfarin (Coumadin) with a PT time greater than 15 seconds
- Heparin within the past 48 hours and an elevated activated partial thromboplastin time (aPTT)
- Platelet count less than 100,000 per mm^3

B. Treatment of ischemic stroke patients with a thrombolytic agent requires a significant neurologic deficit due to stroke. CT scan of the brain must not show acute hemorrhage or a large, already-developing cerebral infarction.

C. Tissue Plasminogen Activator (t-PA) in Ischemic Stroke
  1. T-PA has been demonstrated to be beneficial for patients with ischemic stroke in the carotid or vertebrobasilar circulation. Treatment is beneficial for all types of strokes, including small vessel occlusive disease, large vessel occlusive disease, and cardioembolic stroke.
  2. Patients with an ischemic stroke who are treated with t-PA are 33% more likely to have a normal or near-normal neurologic examination three months after treatment.
  3. Intracerebral hemorrhage occurs in 6.4% of patients who receive t-PA. Patients treated with t-PA who have very large strokes (very severe neurologic deficits) and who already have evidence of a large acute ischemic stroke on CT have an increased risk of intracerebral hemorrhage. However, patients in these two subgroups who receive t-PA are more likely to return to normal.

4. **Dosage and Administration.** The dose of t-PA for acute ischemic stroke is 0.9 mg/kg with a maximum dose of 90 mg. Ten percent of the dose is given as a bolus dose, and the remainder is given over 60 minutes. No heparin or anti-platelet agents (aspirin) should be administered until 24 hours after initiation of t-PA treatment and a 24-hour safety CT has ruled out intracranial hemorrhage.

D. **Blood Pressure Management in Thrombolytic Therapy**
   1. Arterial blood pressure should be kept just below a systolic pressure of 185 mm Hg and a diastolic pressure of 105 mm Hg during the first 24 hours to minimize the risk of intracerebral hemorrhage.
   2. Severe hypertension should be controlled with labetalol, administered at an initial dose of 10 mg IV over 1-2 minutes. The dose may be repeated or doubled every 10-20 minutes if needed or an IV infusion of 2 mg/min may be initiated. If the response is unsatisfactory, then an infusion of sodium nitroprusside starting at a dose of 0.25 mcg/kg/min is recommended.
   3. If the DBP is greater than 140 mmHg, then begin with an infusion of sodium nitroprusside, starting at 0.05 mcg/kg/minute.

V. **General Care**

A. **Blood Pressure**
   1. Acute stroke produces an increase in blood pressure in 80% of patients. Minimal or moderate elevations in blood pressure do not require urgent pharmacological treatment, since there generally is a spontaneous decline in blood pressure over time.
   2. Antihypertensive intervention is not required unless the calculated mean arterial blood pressure is greater than 130 mmHg or the systolic blood pressure is greater than 230 mmHg. Systolic blood pressures between 180-230 mmHg or diastolic pressures 105-120 mmHg may be treated with labetalol hydrochloride and/or nitroprusside. A rapid reduction in the blood pressure is unnecessary and may be harmful. A reduction to systolic blood pressures of 200-230 mmHg and to diastolic pressures of 100-120 mmHg is adequate.

B. **Anticoagulation**
   1. The efficacy of heparin in acute ischemic stroke is not well-established. However, heparin is used commonly in the setting of acute stroke. If thrombolytic therapy (t-PA) has been given, heparin should not be used for 24 hours, and a 24-hour safety CT should be repeated to exclude intracranial hemorrhage.
   2. Heparin has been recommended in: 1) minor strokes; 2) patients who have evolving signs and symptoms; 3) stroke caused by large vessel atherothrombosis; and, 4) cardioembolic stroke. A history of bleeding disorders, recent surgery or trauma, and gastrointestinal bleeding disorders are usually contraindications to the use of heparin. A rectal exam including stool guaiac should be performed prior to the use of heparin. §

Status Epilepticus

Status epilepticus (SE) is defined as continuous seizures lasting at least 5 minutes or 2 or more discrete seizures between which there is incomplete recovery of consciousness. Simple seizures are characterized by focal motor or sensory phenomena, with full preservation of consciousness. Generalized seizures include generalized tonic-clonic seizures. Complex seizures are diagnosed when an alteration in consciousness has occurred.

- I. **Epidemiology**
  - A. SE occurs most often in children and in individuals older than 60 years of age.
  - B. **Causes of generalized seizures** include, in descending order: discontinuation of anticonvulsant drug; alcohol-related seizures; cerebrovascular disease; drug overdose; metabolic disorders; cardiac arrest; and CNS infections, trauma, and cerebral tumors.
  - C. **Toxins and antidotes.** Elicit drugs, theophylline, isoniazid (INH), tricyclic antidepressants, quinolone antibiotics, and sympathomimetics, including cocaine, may precipitate seizures.

Etiology of Status Epilepticus

Status epilepticus in a patient with a history of seizure disorder
- Noncompliance with prescribed medical regimen
- Withdrawal seizures from anticonvulsants
- Breakthrough seizures

New onset seizure disorder presenting with status epilepticus

Status epilepticus secondary to medical, toxicologic, or structural symptoms
- Hypoxic injury: Post-resuscitation
- Stroke syndromes
- Subarachnoid hemorrhage
- Intracranial tumor
- Trauma
- Toxicologic seizures: Theophylline, cocaine, amphetamines isoniazid, alcohol withdrawal
- Metabolic disorders: Hyponatremia, hypernatremia, hypercalcemia, hypomagnesemia, hepatic encephalopathy
- Infectious: Meningitis, brain abscess, encephalitis, CNS cysticercosis or toxoplasmosis

---

- II. **Diagnostic Evaluation**
  - A. **Laboratory evaluation**
    1. **CBC, blood glucose level, serum electrolytes** (sodium, magnesium, calcium), anticonvulsant drug levels, and urinalysis.
    2. **Lumbar puncture** is necessary if meningitis is suspected.
    3. **Toxicologic screening** is indicated in specific situations.
  - B. **CT scan** is indicated if tumor, abscess, hemorrhage, or trauma is suspected, or if the patient has no prior history of seizures.

C. **Electroencephalogram.** An immediate EEG may be required if the patient fails to awaken promptly after clinical termination of the seizures or if there is evidence of subclinical seizure activity.

Differential Diagnosis of Generalized Convulsive Status Epilepticus

Nonepileptic (psychogenic) seizures
Repetitive abnormal posturing (extensor, flexor)
Tetanus
Neuroleptic malignant syndrome
Rigors due to sepsis
Myoclonic jerks
Tremors
Hemiballism
Involuntary movements

III. **Management of Generalized Convulsive Status Epilepticus (GCSE)**
   A. **A history** should be obtained from the patient's family, and a brief physical examination performed.
   B. **Initial stabilization** consists of airway management, 100% oxygen by mask, rapid glucose testing, intravenous access, and cardiac and hemodynamic monitoring.
   C. **Initial Pharmacologic Therapy**
      1. Treatment of status epilepticus should begin with thiamine 100 mg IV push and dextrose 50% water (D5W) 50 mL IV push.
      2. Seizures are treated with lorazepam (Ativan) 0.1 mg/kg IV at 2 mg/min. The same dose may be repeated once. Lorazepam may be given IM if the IV route is unavailable. Lorazepam is preferable to diazepam because of greater efficacy and duration of antiepileptic activity.
      3. Phenytoin or fosphenytoin should be used when benzodiazepines are not effective. The loading dose of phenytoin is 20 mg/kg IV, followed by 4-5 mg/kg/day (100 mg IV q8h or 200 mg IV q12h); maximum rate for each dose is 50 mg/min in normal saline only. An additional loading dose of phenytoin 10 mg/kg may be given if necessary.
      4. **Fosphenytoin (Cerebyx)** is a water soluble prodrug of phenytoin. It may be given IV or IM in normal saline or D5W. The dose of fosphenytoin is expressed in phenytoin equivalents (PE). The loading dose is 20 mg PE/kg IV or IM at 150 mg/min, followed by 100 mg PE IV/IM q8h. The advantages of fosphenytoin are faster loading and greater ease of administration.
   D. **Refractory Status Epilepticus**
      1. Refractory SE is defined as failure of seizure activity to terminate after administration of benzodiazepine and phenytoin, or seizure activity (clinical or EEG) persisting 60 minutes after the onset of the seizure after a benzodiazepine and phenytoin have been given.
      2. Intubation should be accomplished and blood pressure support should be maintained with fluids and pressor agents. EEG monitoring should be maintained.

3. **Midazolam (Versed)** should be administered if seizures continue. Loading dose is 0.2 mg/kg, followed by 0.045 mg/kg/hr. Titrate to 0.6 mg/kg/hr.

4. **Propofol (Diprivan)** may be used if midazolam is ineffective. Loading dose is 1-2 mg/kg, followed by 2 mg/kg/hr, titrate to 10 mg/kg/hr. Adjust dose to achieve seizure-free status on EEG monitoring.

5. **Phenobarbital** may be administered as an alternative to anesthetics if the patient is not hypoxemic or hyperthermic and seizure activity is intermittent (not continuous). The loading dose is 20 mg/kg at 75 mg/min, then 2 mg/kg IV q12h.

6. After seizures have been controlled for 12 hours, infusion of the anesthetic should be slowly reduced and discontinued to allow for neurologic assessment. The drug infusion should be resumed if epileptic activity is observed. §

References

Lowenstein DH, et al. Status epilepticus. N Engl J Med 1998; 338:970-976.

Smith MC, Bleck TP. Techniques for evaluating the cause of coma. Journ Crit Ill 2(12):51-57, 1987.

Rothrock JF, Hart RG. Antithrombotic therapy in cerebrovascular disease. Ann Intern Med 115:885-895, 1991.

Solomon RA, Fink ME. Current strategies for the management of aneurysmal subarachnoid hemorrhage. Arch Neurol 44:769-774, 1987.

Aminoff MJ, Simon RP. Status epilepticus. Am J Med 69:657-665, 1980.

Endocrinologic and Nephrologic Disorders

Naeem Rana, MD
Wenchao Wu, MD

Diabetic Ketoacidosis

In children under 10 years of age, diabetic ketoacidosis causes 70% of diabetes-related deaths. Diabetic ketoacidosis is defined by the triad of hyperglycemia, metabolic acidosis, and ketosis.

I. Clinical Presentation
   A. Diabetes is newly diagnosed in 20% of cases of diabetic ketoacidosis. The remainder of cases occur in known diabetics in whom ketosis develops because of a precipitating factor, such as infection or noncompliance with insulin.
   B. Symptoms of DKA include polyuria, polydipsia, fatigue, nausea, and vomiting, developing over 1 to 2 days. Abdominal pain is prominent in 25%.
   C. Physical Exam
      1. Patients are typically flushed, tachycardic, and tachypneic. Kussmaul's respiration, with deep breathing and air hunger, occurs when the serum pH is between 7.0 and 7.24.
      2. A fruity odor on the breath indicates the presence of acetone, a by-product of diabetic ketoacidosis.
      3. Fever is seldom present even though infection is common. Hypothermia and hypotension may also occur. Eighty percent of patients with diabetic ketoacidosis have altered mental status. Most are awake but confused; 10% are comatose.
   D. Laboratory Findings
      1. Serum glucose level >250 mg/dL
      2. pH <7.35
      3. Bicarbonate level below normal with an elevated anion gap
      4. Presence of ketones in the serum

Indications for Hospital Admission of Patients with Diabetic Ketoacidosis

Hyperglycemia (glucose >250 mg/dL)
Arterial pH <7.35, or venous pH <7.30, or serum bicarbonate <15 mEq/L
Ketonuria, ketonemia, or both

II. Differential Diagnosis
   A. Differential Diagnosis of Ketosis-Causing Conditions
      1. **Alcoholic ketoacidosis** does not cause an elevated serum glucose. Alcoholic ketoacidosis occurs with heavy drinking and vomiting.
      2. Starvation ketosis occurs after 24 hours without food and is not usually confused with DKA because glucose and serum pH are normal.

B. Differential Diagnosis of Acidosis-Causing Conditions
1. **Metabolic acidoses** are divided into increased anion gap (>14 mEq/L) and normal anion gap (anion gap is determined by subtracting the sum of chloride plus bicarbonate from sodium).
2. **Anion gap acidoses** can be caused by any of the ketoacidoses, including DKA, lactic acidosis, uremia, salicylate or methanol poisoning.
3. **Non-anion gap acidoses** are associated with a normal glucose level and absent serum ketones. Non-anion gap acidoses are caused by renal or gastrointestinal electrolyte losses.

C. Hyperglycemia caused by hyperosmolar nonketotic coma occurs in
patients with type II diabetes with severe hyperglycemia. Patients are usually elderly and have a precipitating illness. Glucose level is markedly elevated (>600 mg/dL), osmolarity is increased, and ketosis is minimal.

III. Treatment of Diabetic Ketoacidosis
A. Fluid Resuscitation
1. Fluid deficits average 5 liters or 50 mL/kg. Resuscitation consists of 1 liter of normal saline over the first hour and a second liter over the second and third hours. Thereafter, ½ normal saline should be infused at 250 mL/hr.
2. When the glucose level decreases to 250 mg/dL, 5% dextrose should be added to the replacement fluids to prevent hypoglycemia. If the glucose level declines rapidly, 10% dextrose should be infused, along with regular insulin, until the anion gap normalizes.

B. Insulin
1. Insulin is infused at 0.1 U/kg per hour. The biologic half life of IV insulin is less than 20 minutes. The insulin infusion should be adjusted each hour so that the glucose decline does not exceed 100 mg/dL per hour.
2. When the bicarbonate level is greater than 20 mEq/L and the anion gap is less than 16 mEq/L, the insulin infusion rate may be decreased.

C. Potassium
1. The most common preventable cause of death in patients with DKA is hypokalemia. The typical deficit is between 300 and 600 mEq.
2. Potassium chloride should be started when fluid therapy is started. In most patients, the initial rate of potassium replacement is 20 mEq/h, but hypokalemia requires more aggressive replacement (40 mEq/h).
3. All patients should receive potassium replacement, except for those with renal failure, no urine output, or an initial serum potassium level greater than 6.0 mEq/L.

D. Sodium
1. Patients with diabetic ketoacidosis sometimes have a low serum sodium level because the high level of glucose has a dilutional effect. For every 100 mg/dL that glucose is elevated, the sodium level should be assumed to be higher than the measured value by 1.6 mEq/L.
2. Frequently, patients have an initial serum sodium greater than 150 mEq/L, indicating severe dehydration. For these patients, initial rehydration fluid should consist of ½ normal saline.

E. Phosphate
1. Diabetic ketoacidosis depletes phosphate stores.

    2. Serum phosphate level should be checked after 4 hours of treatment. If it is below 1.5 mg/dL, potassium phosphate should be added to the IV solution.

F. Bicarbonate therapy is not required unless the arterial pH value is 7.0 or lower. For a pH of <7.0, intravenous administration of 50 mEq/L of sodium bicarbonate is recommended.

G. Additional Therapies

    1. A nasogastric tube should be inserted in semiconscious patients to protect against aspiration.

    2. Deep vein thrombosis prophylaxis with subcutaneous heparin should be provided for patients who are elderly, unconscious, or severely hyperosmolar (5,000 U every 12 hours).

IV.Monitoring of Therapy

A. Serum bicarbonate level and anion gap should be monitored to determine the effectiveness of insulin therapy.

B. Glucose levels should be check glucose level at 1-2 hour intervals during IV insulin administration.

C. Electrolyte levels should be assessed every 2 hours for the first 6-8 hours, and then q4h. Phosphorus and magnesium levels should be checked after 4 hours of treatment.

D. Plasma and urine ketones are helpful in diagnosing diabetic ketoacidosis, but are not necessary during therapy.

V. Determining the Underlying Cause

A. Infection is the underlying cause of diabetic ketoacidosis in 50% of cases. Infection of the urinary tract, respiratory tract, skin, sinuses, ears, or teeth should be sought. Fever is unusual in diabetic ketoacidosis and indicates infection when present. If infection is suspected, antibiotics should be promptly initiated.

B. Omission of insulin doses (common in adolescents) is often a precipitating factor.

C. Myocardial infarction, ischemic stroke, and abdominal catastrophes may precipitate DKA.

VI.Initiation of Subcutaneous Insulin

A. When the serum bicarbonate and anion gap levels are normal, subcutaneous regular insulin can be started.

B. Intravenous and subcutaneous administration of insulin should overlap to avoid redevelopment of ketoacidosis. The intravenous infusion may be stopped 1 hour after the first subcutaneous injection insulin.

C. Estimation of Subcutaneous Insulin Requirements

    1. Multiply the final insulin infusion rate times 24 hours. Two thirds of the total dose is given in the morning as two thirds NPH and one third regular insulin. The remaining one third of the total dose is given before supper as one half NPH and one half regular insulin.

    2. Subsequent doses should be adjusted according to the patient's blood glucose response. §

Acute Renal Failure

Acute renal failure is defined as a sudden decrease in renal function sufficient to increase the concentration of nitrogenous wastes in the blood. It is characterized by an increasing BUN and creatinine.

I. Clinical Presentation of Acute Renal Failure

A. **Oliguria** is a common indicator of acute renal failure, and it is marked by a decrease in urine output to less than 30 mL/h. Acute renal failure may be oliguric (<500 L/day) or nonoliguric (>30 mL/h). Anuria (<100 mL/day) does not usually occur in renal failure, and its presence suggests obstruction or a vascular cause.

B. Acute renal failure may less commonly be manifest by encephalopathy, volume overload, pericarditis, bleeding, anemia, hyperkalemia, hyperphosphatemia, hypocalcemia, and metabolic acidemia.

II. Clinical Causes of Renal Failure

A. **Prerenal Insult**

1. Prerenal insult is the most common cause of acute renal failure, accounting for 70% of cases. Prerenal failure is usually caused by reduced renal perfusion pressure secondary to extracellular fluid volume loss (diarrhea, diuresis, GI hemorrhage), or secondary to extracellular fluid sequestration (pancreatitis, sepsis), inadequate cardiac output, renal vasoconstriction (sepsis, liver disease, drugs), or inadequate fluid intake or replacement.

2. Most patients with prerenal azotemia have oliguria, a history of large fluid losses (vomiting, diarrhea, burns), and evidence of intravascular volume depletion (thirst, weight loss, orthostatic hypotension, tachycardia, flat neck veins, dry mucous membranes). Patients with congestive heart failure may have total body volume excess (distended neck veins, pulmonary and pedal edema) but still have compromised renal perfusion and prerenal azotemia because of diminished cardiac output.

3. The causes of prerenal failure are usually reversible if recognized and treated early; otherwise, prolonged renal hypoperfusion can lead to acute tubular necrosis and permanent renal insufficiency.

B. **Intrarenal Insult**

1. **Acute tubular necrosis (ATN)** is the most common intrinsic renal disease leading to ARF.

   a. Prolonged renal hypoperfusion is the most common cause of ATN.

   b. **Nephrotoxic agents** (aminoglycosides, heavy metals, radiocontrast media, ethylene glycol) represent exogenous nephrotoxins. ATN may also occur as a result of endogenous nephrotoxins, such as intratubular pigments (hemoglobinuria), intratubular proteins (myeloma), and intratubular crystals (uric acid).

2. **Acute interstitial nephritis (AIN)** is an Allergic reaction secondary to drugs (NSAIDs, β-lactams, and many other drugs).

3. **Arteriolar injury** occurs secondary to hypertension, vasculitis, microangiopathic disorders.

4. **Glomerulonephritis** secondary to immunologically mediated inflammation may cause intrarenal damage.

C. **Postrenal insult** results from obstruction of urine flow. Postrenal insult is the least common cause of acute renal failure, accounting for 10%.

1. Postrenal insult may be caused by extra-renal obstructive uropathy secondary to prostate cancer, benign prostatic hypertrophy, or renal calculi occlusion of the bladder outlet.
2. Postrenal insult may be caused by intra-renal obstruction of the distal tubules by amyloidosis, uric acid crystals, multiple myeloma, or by methotrexate or acyclovir.

III. Clinical evaluation of acute renal failure

A. **Initial evaluation** of renal failure should determine whether the cause is decreased renal perfusion, obstructed urine flow, or disorders involving the renal parenchyma. Recent clinical events and drug therapy should be reviewed, including volume status (orthostatic pulse, blood pressure, fluid intake and output, daily weights, hemodynamic parameters), nephrotoxic medications, and pattern of urine output.

B. **Prerenal azotemia** is likely when there is a history of heart failure or extracellular fluid volume loss or depletion.

C. **Postrenal azotemia** is suggested by a history of decreased size or force of the urine stream, anuria, flank pain, hematuria or pyuria, or cancer of the bladder, prostate or pelvis. Anuria usually results from obstructive uropathy; occasionally anuria indicates cessation of renal blood flow or rapidly progressive glomerulonephritis.

D. **Intrarenal insult** is suggested by a history of prolonged volume depletion (often post-surgical), pigmenturia, hemolysis, rhabdomyolysis, or nephrotoxins. Intrarenal insult is suggested by recent radiocontrast, aminoglycoside use, or vascular catheterization. Interstitial nephritis may be implicated by a history of medication rash, fever, or arthralgias. Urinary studies may reveal hematuria, sterile pyuria, eosinophiluria, mild proteinuria (<2 g/24 h) and, rarely, white blood cell casts. NSAID-induced acute interstitial nephritis occurs most often with the use of ibuprofen, fenoprofen, and naproxen.

E. **Chronic renal failure** is suggested by the presence of a disease known to cause chronic renal insufficiency (diabetes mellitus). The presence of normochromic normocytic anemia, hypercalcemia, and hyperphosphatemia also suggests chronic renal insufficiency.

IV. Physical Examination

A. Cardiac output, volume status, bladder size, and systemic disease manifestations should be assessed.

B. **Prerenal azotemia** is suggested by impaired cardiac output (neck vein distention, pulmonary rales, pedal edema). Volume depletion is suggested by orthostatic blood pressure changes, weight loss, low urine output, or diuretic use.

C. **Flank, suprapubic, or abdominal masses** may indicate an obstructive cause.

D. **Skin rash** may suggests drug-induced interstitial nephritis; palpable purpura suggests vasculitis; nonpalpable purpura suggests thrombotic thrombocytopenic purpura or hemolytic-uremic syndrome, all of which are compatible with intrarenal kidney failure.

E. **Bladder catheterization** is useful to rule out suspected bladder outlet obstruction. A residual volume of more than 100 mL suggests bladder outlet obstruction.

F. **Central venous monitoring** is used to measure cardiac output and left ventricular filling pressure if prerenal failure is suspected.

V. Laboratory Evaluation
A. Spot Urine Sodium Concentration
1. Spot urine sodium can help distinguish between prerenal azotemia and acute tubular necrosis.
2. Prerenal failure causes increased reabsorption of salt and water and will manifest as a low spot urine sodium concentration <20 mEq/L and a low fractional sodium excretion <1%, and a urine/plasma creatinine >40. Fractional Excretion of Sodium (%) = ([urine sodium/plasma sodium] ÷ [urine creatinine/plasma creatinine] x 100). FENA may be less reliable if the patient is elderly, received diuretics, or has pre-existing renal disease, acute glomerulonephritis, or cirrhosis.
3. If tubular necrosis is the cause, the spot urine concentration will be >40 mEq/L, and fractional excretion of sodium will be >1% because necrosed tubules do not efficiently reabsorb sodium. Urine spot sodium is less reliable if loop diuretics have been used in the preceding 24 hours.
4. A urine/plasma creatinine <20 is consistent with renal failure.

B. Urinalysis
1. **Normal urine sediment** is a strong indicator of prerenal azotemia or may be an indicator of obstructive uropathy.
2. **Hematuria, pyuria, or crystals** may be associated with postrenal obstructive azotemia.
3. **Abundant cells, casts, or protein** suggests an intrarenal disorder.
4. **Red cells** alone may indicate vascular disorders; RBC casts and abundant protein suggest glomerular disease (glomerulonephritis).
5. **White cell casts and eosinophilic casts** indicate interstitial nephritis.
6. **Renal epithelial cell casts and pigmented granular casts** are associated acute tubular necrosis.

C. Ultrasound
is useful for evaluation of suspected postrenal obstruction (nephrolithiasis) after bladder outlet obstruction has been ruled out by catheterization. The presence of small (<10 cm in length), scarred kidneys is diagnostic of chronic renal insufficiency.

D. Renal biopsy:
If clinical findings make acute tubular necrosis or prerenal azotemia unlikely, further evaluation and biopsy are indicated.

VI. Management of Acute Renal Failure
A. Reversible disorders, such as obstruction, should be excluded, and hypovolemia should be corrected with volume replacement. Cardiac output should be maintained.
B. In critically ill patients, physical examination and chest film are often inadequate guides to hemodynamic status; therefore, a pulmonary artery catheter should be used for monitoring.
C. **Extracellular Fluid Volume Expansion.** Infusion of a 1-2 liter crystalloid fluid bolus may confirm suspected volume-depleted, prerenal azotemia.
D. If the patient remains oliguric despite euvolemia, IV diuretics may be administered. Nonoliguric acute tubular necrosis is associated with a more favorable prognostic outcome than oliguric renal failure, and metabolic complications are less likely.
1. A large single dose of furosemide (100-200 mg) may be administered intravenously to promote diuresis. If urine flow is not improved, the dose of furosemide may be doubled or given in combination with metolazone (Zaroxolyn). Furosemide may be repeated in 2 hours, or

a continuous IV infusion of 10-40 mg/hr (max 1000 mg/day) may be used.

E. The dosage or dosing intervals of renally excreted drugs should be modified. Drug levels, blood cell count, electrolytes, creatinine, calcium, and phosphorus levels should be monitored.

F. **Hyperkalemia** is the most immediately life-threatening complication of renal failure. Serum potassium values greater than 6.5 mEq/L may lead to arrhythmias and cardiac arrest. Potassium should be removed from IV solutions. Hyperkalemia may be treated with sodium polystyrene sulfonate (Kayexalate), 30-60 gm PO/PR every 4-6 hours.

G. **Hyperphosphatemia** can be controlled with aluminum hydroxide given with meals to bind dietary phosphorus. Antacids that contain magnesium are contraindicated.

H. **Fluids.** After normal volume has been restored, fluid intake should be reduced to an amount equal to urinary and other losses plus insensible losses of 300-500 mL/day. In oliguric patients, daily fluid intake may need to be restricted to less than 1 L.

I. **Nutritional Therapy.** A renal diet consisting of daily high biologic value protein intake of 0.5 gm/kg/d, sodium 2 g, potassium 40-60 mg/day, and at least 35 kcal/kg of nonprotein calories is recommended. Phosphorus should be restricted to 800 mg/day

J. **Dialysis.** Indications for dialysis include uremic pericarditis, severe hyperkalemia, pulmonary edema, persistent severe metabolic acidosis (pH less than 7.2), and symptomatic uremia. §

Hyperkalemia

Ninety-eight percent of body K is intracellular. Only 2% of total body potassium, about 70 mEq, is in the extracellular fluid with the normal concentration of 3.5-5 mEq/L.

I. **Pathophysiology of Potassium Homeostasis**
   A. The normal upper limit of plasma K is 5-5.5 mEq/L, with a mean K level of 4.3.
   B. **External Potassium Balance.** Normal dietary K intake is 1-1.5 mEq/kg in the form of vegetables and meats. The kidney is the primary organ for preserving external K balance, excreting 90% of the daily K burden.
   C. **Internal potassium balance**, potassium transfer to and from tissues, is affected by insulin, acid-base status, catecholamines, aldosterone, plasma osmolality, cellular necrosis, glucagon, and drugs.

II. **Clinical Disorders of External Potassium Balance**
   A. **Chronic Renal Failure.** The kidney is able to excrete the normal dietary intake of potassium until the glomerular filtration rate falls below 10 cc/minute or until urine output falls below 1 L/day. Renal failure is advanced before hyperkalemia occurs.
   B. **Impaired Renal Tubular Function.** Renal diseases may cause hyperkalemia, and the renal tubular acidosis caused by these conditions may worsen hyperkalemia.
   C. **Primary Adrenal Insufficiency (Addison's disease)** is now a rare cause of hyperkalemia.
      1. **Diagnosis** is indicated by the combination of hyperkalemia and hyponatremia and is confirmed by a low aldosterone and a low plasma

cortisol level that does not respond to adrenocorticotropic hormone treatment.

   2. Treatment consists of glucocorticoid and mineralocorticoid agents and volume replacement with normal saline.

D. **Drugs** that may cause hyperkalemia include nonsteroidal anti-inflammatory drugs, angiotensin-converting enzyme inhibitors, cyclosporine, and potassium-sparing diuretics. Hyperkalemia is especially common when these drugs are given to patients at risk for hyperkalemia (diabetics, renal failure, hyporeninemic hypoaldosteronism, advanced age).

E. **Excessive Potassium Intake**
   1. Long-term potassium supplementation results in hyperkalemia most often when an underlying impairment in renal excretion already exists.
   2. Oral ingestion of 1 mEq/kg may increase the serum K level by 1 mEq/L an hour afterward in normal individuals. Intravenous administration of 0.5 mEq/kg over 1 hour increases serum levels by 0.6 mEq/L. Hyperkalemia often results when infusions of greater than 40 mEq/hour are given.

III. Clinical Disorders of Internal Potassium Balance

A. **Diabetic patients** are at particular risk for severe hyperkalemia because of renal insufficiency and hyporeninemic hypoaldosteronism.

B. **Systemic acidosis** reduces renal excretion of potassium and moves potassium out of cells, resulting in hyperkalemia.

C. **Endogenous potassium release** from muscle injury, tumor lysis, or chemotherapy may elevate serum potassium.

IV. Manifestations of Hyperkalemia

A. Hyperkalemia, unless severe, is usually asymptomatic. The effect of hyperkalemia on the heart becomes significant above 6 mEq/L. As levels increase, the initial ECG change is tall peaked T waves. The QT interval is normal or diminished.

B. As K levels rise further, the PR interval becomes prolonged, then the P wave amplitude decreases. The QRS complex widens into a sine wave pattern, with subsequent cardiac standstill.

C. At serum K levels of >7 mEq/L, muscle weakness may lead to a flaccid paralysis that spares cranial nerve function. Sensory abnormalities, impaired speech, and respiratory arrest may follow.

V. Pseudohyperkalemia

A. Potassium may be falsely elevated by hemolysis during phlebotomy, when K is released from ischemic muscle distal to a tourniquet, and because of erythrocyte fragility disorders.

B. Falsely high laboratory measurement of serum potassium may occur in normokalemic subjects who have a markedly elevated platelet (>10^6 platelet/mm^3) or white blood cell (>50,000/mm^3) counts.

VI. Diagnostic Approach to Hyperkalemia

A. The serum K level should be repeat tested to rule out laboratory error. If significant thrombocytosis or leukocytosis is present, a plasma potassium level should be determined.

B. Measure 24 hour urine output, urinary K excretion, blood urea nitrogen, and serum creatinine. Renal K retention is diagnosed when urinary K excretion is less than 20 mEq/day.

C. High urinary K, excretion of >20 mEq/day, is indicative of excessive K intake as the cause.

VII. Renal Hyperkalemia

 A. If urinary K excretion is low and urine output is in the oliguric range and creatinine clearance is lower than 20 cc/minute, renal failure is the probable cause. Prerenal azotemia resulting from volume depletion must be ruled out because the hyperkalemia will respond to volume restoration.

 B. When urinary K excretion is low, yet blood urea nitrogen and creatinine levels are not elevated and urine volume is at least 1 L daily and renal sodium excretion is adequate (about 20 mEq/day), then either a defect in the secretion of renin or aldosterone or tubular resistance to aldosterone is likely. Low plasma renin and aldosterone levels, will confirm the diagnosis of hyporeninemic hypoaldosteronism. Addison's disease is suggested by a low serum cortisol, and the diagnosis is confirmed with a ACTH (Cortrosyn) stimulation test.

 C. When inadequate K excretion is not caused by hypoaldosteronism, a tubular defect in K clearance is suggested. Urinary tract obstruction, renal transplant, lupus, or a medication should be considered.

VIII. Extrarenal Hyperkalemia

 A. When hyperkalemia occurs along with high urinary K excretion of >20 mEq/day, excessive intake of K is the cause. Potassium excess in IV fluids, diet, or medication should be sought. A concomitant underlying renal defect in K excretion is also likely to be present.

 B. Blood sugar should be measured to rule out insulin deficiency; blood pH and serum bicarbonate should be measured to rule out acidosis.

 C. Endogenous sources of K, such as tissue necrosis, hypercatabolism, hematoma, gastrointestinal bleeding, or intravascular hemolysis should be excluded.

IX. Management of Hyperkalemia

 A. Acute Treatment of Hyperkalemia

 1. Calcium Chloride or gluconate

 a. If the electrocardiogram shows loss of P waves or widening of QRS complexes, calcium chloride should be given IV; calcium reduces the cell membrane threshold potential but will not lower the potassium level.

 b. Calcium gluconate 10% should be given as 2-3 ampules over 5 minutes. In patients with circulatory compromise, 1 ampule of calcium chloride IV should be given over 3 minutes.

 c. If the serum K level is greater than 7 mEq/L, calcium should be given because of imminent cardiac toxicity. If digitalis intoxication is suspected, calcium must be given cautiously. Coexisting hyponatremia should be treated with hypertonic saline.

 2. Insulin

 a. If the only ECG abnormalities are peaked T waves and the serum level is under 7 mEq/L, treatment should begin with insulin (regular insulin, 5-10 U by IV push) with 50% dextrose water (D50W) 50 mL IV push (unless the blood sugar is already substantially elevated).

 b. Repeated insulin doses of 10 U and glucose can be given every 15 minutes for maximal effect.

 3. Sodium Bicarbonate

 a. Bicarbonate promotes cellular uptake of K, and it should be given as 1-2 ampules (50-mEq/ampule) IV push.

 b. Bicarbonate should be avoided if severe heart failure or hypernatremia. If the serum calcium is low (as in uremic acidosis), calcium should also be given in a separate IV line to avoid hypocalcemic tetany during alkali therapy.

4. **Potassium Elimination Measures**
   a. Furosemide (Lasix) 100 mg IV should be given immediately to promote kaliuresis; normal saline may be added to avoid volume depletion.
   b. Sodium polystyrene sulfonate (Kayexalate) is a cation exchange resin that binds to potassium in the lower GI tract. Dosage is 30-60 gm premixed with sorbitol 20% PO/PR.
   c. Emergent hemodialysis for hyperkalemia is not usually necessary, even in renal failure. §

Hypokalemia

Hypokalemia is characterized by a serum K concentration of less than 3.5 mEq/L. Ninety-eight percent of K is intracellular.

I. **Pathophysiology of Hypokalemia**

A. **Cellular Redistribution of Potassium.** Hypokalemia may result from the intracellular shift of potassium by insulin, beta-2 agonist drugs, stress induced catecholamine release, thyrotoxic periodic paralysis, and alkalosis-induced shift (metabolic or respiratory).

B. **Nonrenal Potassium Loss**
   1. Gastrointestinal loss can be caused by diarrhea, laxative abuse, villous adenoma, biliary drainage, enteric fistula, clay ingestion, potassium binding resin ingestion, or nasogastric suction.
   2. Sweating, prolonged low potassium ingestion, hemodialysis and peritoneal dialysis may also cause nonrenal potassium loss.

C. **Renal Potassium Loss**
   1. **Hypertensive High Renin States.** Malignant hypertension, renal artery stenosis, renin-producing tumors.
   2. **Hypertensive Low Renin, High Aldosterone States.** Primary hyperaldosteronism (adenoma or hyperplasia).
   3. **Hypertensive Low Renin, Low Aldosterone States.** Congenital adrenal hyperplasia (11 or 17 hydroxylase deficiency), Cushing's syndrome or disease, exogenous mineralocorticoids (Florinef, licorice, chewing tobacco), Liddle's syndrome.
   4. **Normotensive States**
      a. **Metabolic Acidosis.** Renal tubular acidosis (type I or II)
      b. **Metabolic Alkalosis (urine chloride <10 mEq/day).** Vomiting
      c. **Metabolic Alkalosis (urine chloride >10 mEq/day).** Bartter's syndrome, diuretics, magnesium depletion, normotensive hyperaldosteronism
   5. **Drugs** associated with potassium loss include amphotericin B, ticarcillin, piperacillin, and loop diuretics.

II. **Clinical Effects of Hypokalemia**

A. **Cardiac Effects**. The most lethal consequence of hypokalemia is cardiac arrhythmias. Electrocardiographic effects include depressed ST segments, decreased T-wave amplitude, U waves, and a prolonged QT-U interval.

    B. Musculoskeletal Effects. The initial manifestation of K depletion is muscle weakness, which can lead to paralysis. In severe cases, respiratory muscle paralysis may occur.

    C. Gastrointestinal Effects. Nausea, vomiting, constipation, and paralytic ileus may develop.

III. Diagnostic Evaluation

    A. The 24-hour urinary potassium excretion should be measured.

    B. If >20 mEq/day, excessive urinary K loss is the cause. If <20 mEq/d, low K intake, or non-urinary K loss is the cause.

    C. In patients with excessive renal K loss and hypertension, plasma renin and aldosterone should be measured to differentiate adrenal from non-adrenal causes of hyperaldosteronism.

    D. If hypertension is absent and patient is acidotic, renal tubular acidosis should be considered.

    E. If hypertension is absent and serum pH is normal to alkalotic, a high urine chloride (>10 mEq/d) suggests hypokalemia secondary to diuretics or Bartter's syndrome. A low urine chloride (<10 mEq/d) suggests vomiting.

IV. Emergency Treatment of Hypokalemia

    A. Indications for Urgent Replacement. Electrocardiographic abnormalities consistent with severe K depletion, myocardial infarction, hypoxia, digitalis intoxication, marked muscle weakness, or respiratory muscle paralysis.

    B. Intravenous Potassium Therapy

        1. Intravenous KCL is usually used unless concomitant hypophosphatemia is present (diabetic ketoacidosis), where potassium phosphate is indicated.

        2. The maximal rate of intravenous K replacement is 30 mEq/hour. The K concentration of IV fluids should be 80 mEq/L or less if given via a peripheral vein. Frequent monitoring of serum K and constant electrocardiographic monitoring is recommended when depleted potassium levels are being replaced.

V. Non-Emergent Treatment of Hypokalemia

    A. Attempts should be made to normalize K levels if <3.5 mEq/L.

    B. Oral supplementation is significantly safer than IV. The liquid formulation is preferred due to rapid oral absorption over 30-60 minutes, compared to sustained release formulations, which are absorbed over several hours. Micro-encapsulated and sustained-release forms of KCL are less likely to induce gastrointestinal disturbances than are wax-matrix tablets or liquid preparations.

        1. KCL elixir 20-40 mEq qd-tid PO after meals.

        2. Micro-K, 10 mEq tabs, 2-3 tabs tid PO after meals (40-100 mEq/d). §

Hypomagnesemia

Magnesium deficiency occurs in up to 11% of hospitalized patients. The most common diagnoses in patients with acute magnesium depletion are malignancy, chronic obstructive pulmonary disease, and alcoholism. The normal range of serum magnesium is 1.5 to 2.0 (±0.2) mEq/L, which is maintained by the kidney, intestine, and bone.

I. **Pathophysiology**
   A. **Decreased Magnesium Intake.** Protein-calorie malnutrition, prolonged parenteral (Mg-free) fluid administration, and catabolic illness are common causes of hypomagnesemia.
   B. **Gastrointestinal Losses of Magnesium.** Gastrointestinal losses of magnesium may result from prolonged nasogastric suction, laxative abuse, pancreatitis, extensive small bowel resection, short bowel syndromes, biliary and bowel fistulas, enteropathies, cholestatic liver disease, and malabsorption syndromes.
   C. **Renal Losses of Magnesium**
      1. Renal loss of magnesium may occur secondary to renal tubular acidosis, glomerulonephritis, interstitial nephritis, or acute tubular necrosis.
      2. Hyperthyroidism, hypercalcemia, and hypophosphatemia may cause magnesium loss.
      3. **Agents that enhance magnesium renal excretion** include alcohol, loop and thiazide diuretics, amphotericin B, aminoglycosides, cisplatin, pentamidine, and colony stimulating factor therapy.
   D. **Alterations in Magnesium Distribution**
      1. Redistribution of circulating magnesium occurs by extracellular to intracellular shifts, sequestration, hungry bone syndrome, or by acute administration of glucose, insulin, or amino acids.
      2. Magnesium depletion occurs during severe pancreatitis, large quantities of parenteral fluids, and pancreatitis-induced sequestration of magnesium.

II. **Clinical Manifestations of Hypomagnesemia**
   A. **Cardiovascular.** Ventricular tachycardia, ventricular fibrillation, atrial fibrillation, multifocal atrial tachycardia, ventricular ectopic beats, hypertension, enhancement of digoxin-induced dysrhythmias, and cardiomyopathies.
   B. **Neuromuscular findings** may include positive Chvostek's and Trousseau's signs, tremors, myoclonic jerks, seizures and, eventually, coma.
   C. **ECG Changes** may include a spectrum of ventricular arrhythmias (extrasystoles, tachycardia) and atrial arrhythmias (atrial fibrillation, supraventricular tachycardia), as well as torsades de pointes. Prolonged PR and QT intervals, ST segment depression, T wave inversions, wide QRS complexes, and tall T waves may occur.
   D. **Concomitant electrolyte abnormalities** of sodium, potassium, calcium, or phosphate are common.

III. **Clinical Evaluation**
   A. Hypomagnesemia is diagnosed when the serum magnesium is less than 0.7-0.8 mMol/L. Symptoms of magnesium deficiency occur when the serum magnesium concentration is less than 0.5 mMol/L. 24-hour urine collection for magnesium is the first step in the evaluation of hypomagnesemia. In hypomagnesemic states, because of renal magnesium loss, magnesium excretion exceeds 24 mg/day.
   B. Low urinary magnesium excretion (<1 mMol/day), with concomitant serum hypomagnesemia, suggests magnesium deficiency due to decreased intake, nonrenal losses, or redistribution of magnesium.

IV. Treatment of Hypomagnesemia

A. Asymptomatic Magnesium Deficiency

1. In hospitalized patients, the daily magnesium requirements can be provided through either a balanced diet, as oral magnesium supplements (0.36-0.46 mEq/kg/day), or 16-30 mEq/day in a parenteral nutrition formulation.

2. Magnesium oxide is better absorbed and less likely to cause diarrhea than magnesium sulfate. Magnesium oxide preparations include Mag-Ox 400 (240 mg elemental magnesium per 400 mg tablet), Uro-Mag (84 mg elemental magnesium per 400 mg tablet), and magnesium chloride (Slo-Mag) 64 mg/tab, 1-2 tabs bid.

B. Symptomatic Magnesium Deficiency

1. Serum magnesium ≤ 0.5 mMol/L requires IV magnesium repletion with electrocardiographic and respiratory monitoring.

2. Magnesium sulfate 1-6 gm of in 500 mL of D5W can be infused IV at 1 gm/hr. An additional 6-9 gm of $MgSO_4$ should be provided as intermittent bolus therapy or by continuous infusion over the next 24 hours. Parenteral $MgSO_4$ (4 mMol/g) is more frequently used than $MgCl_2$.

3. States of severe magnesium deficiency may require additional therapy over a number of days because of slow repletion of cellular magnesium stores.

4. Polymorphic ventricular tachycardia (Torsade de Pointes) may be caused by hypomagnesemia. It is characterized by polymorphic VT with long QT intervals. Treatment consists of $MgSO_4$ 2-4 gm IV over 5-10 min, followed by 8-12 gm infused over 24 hours. §

Hypermagnesemia

Serum magnesium has a normal range of 0.8-1.2 mMol/L. Magnesium homeostasis is regulated by renal and gastrointestinal mechanisms. Hypermagnesemia is usually iatrogenic and is frequently seen in conjunction with renal insufficiency.

I. Clinical Evaluation of Hypermagnesemia

A. Causes of Hypermagnesemia

1. **Renal.** Creatinine clearance <30 mL/minute.

2. **Nonrenal.** Excessive use of magnesium cathartics, especially with renal failure; iatrogenic overtreatment with magnesium sulfate.

3. **Less Common Causes of Mild Hypermagnesemia.** Hyperparathyroidism, Addison's disease, hypocalciuric hypercalcemia, and lithium therapy.

B. Hypermagnesemia is commonly caused by overzealous replacement of magnesium, inadequate adjustment of magnesium dosage for renal insufficiency, and overuse of magnesium-containing cathartics.

1. **Cardiovascular Manifestations of Hypermagnesemia**

   a. **Lower levels of hypermagnesemia <10 mEq/L.** Delayed interventricular conduction, first-degree heart block, prolongation of the Q-T interval.

      (1) Sever, symptomatic hypermagnesemia should be treated with 10% calcium gluconate (10-20 mL) over 10 minutes.

Mechanical ventilation is indicated for respiratory failure and temporary pacemaker for bradycardia.

(2) Hemodialysis is definitive treatment.

(3) In absence of renal failure, normal saline with 2 gm calcium gluconate per liter can be given at 150-200 mL/hr to promote magnesium excretion. Loop diuretics can be used after volume expansion with saline.

b. Levels greater than 10 mEq/L. Low grade heart block progressing to complete heart block and asystole occurs at levels greater than 12.5 mMol/L (>6.25 mMol/L).

2. **Neuromuscular Effects**

a. Hyporeflexia occurs at a magnesium level >4 mEq/L (>2 mMol/L); an early sign of magnesium toxicity is diminution of deep tendon reflexes caused by neuromuscular blockade.

b. Respiratory depression due to respiratory muscle paralysis, somnolence and coma occur at levels >13 mEq/L (6.5 mMol/L).

c. Hypermagnesemia should always be considered when these symptoms occur in patients with renal failure, in those receiving therapeutic magnesium, and in laxative abuse.

II. Treatment of Hypermagnesemia

A. **Asymptomatic, Hemodynamically Stable Patients**. Moderate hypermagnesemia can be managed by elimination of intake and maintenance of renal magnesium clearance.

B. **Severe Hypermagnesemia**

1. Furosemide 20-40 mg IV q3-4h should be given as needed. Saline diuresis should be initiated with 0.9% saline, infused at 150 cc/h to replace urine loss.

2. If ECG abnormalities (peaked T waves, loss of P waves, or widened QRS complexes) or if respiratory depression is present, IV calcium gluconate should be given as 1-3 ampules (10% sln, 1 gm per 10 mL amp), added to saline infusate. Calcium gluconate can be infused to reverse acute cardiovascular toxicity or respiratory failure as 15 mg/kg over a 4-hour period.

3. Parenteral insulin and glucose can be given to shift magnesium into cells. Dialysis is necessary for patients who have severe hypermagnesemia after stabilization of the ECG findings. §

Disorders of Water and Sodium Balance

I. **Pathophysiology of Water and Sodium Balance**

A. Volitional intake of water is regulated by thirst.

B. Maintenance intake of water is the amount of water sufficient to offset obligatory losses.

C. **Maintenance Water Needs.**
   = 100 mL/kg for first 10 kg of body weight
   + 50 mL/kg for next 10 kg
   + 20 mL/kg for weight greater than 20 kg

D. **Clinical Signs of Hyponatremia.** Confusion, agitation, lethargy, seizures, and coma. The rate of change of sodium concentration during onset of hyponatremia is more important in causing symptoms than is the absolute concentration of sodium.

E. Pseudohyponatremia

1. A marked elevation of the blood glucose creates an osmotic gradient that pulls water from cells into the extracellular fluid, diluting the extracellular sodium. The contribution of hyperglycemia to hyponatremia can be estimated using the following formula:

   Expected change in serum sodium = (Serum glucose - 100) x 0.016

2. Marked elevation of plasma solids (lipids or protein) can also result in erroneous hyponatremia because of laboratory inaccuracy. The percentage of plasma water can be estimated with the following formula:

   % plasma water = 100 - [0.01 x lipids (mg/dL)] - [0.73 x protein (g/dL)]

II. Diagnostic Evaluation of Hyponatremia

A. Pseudohyponatremia should be excluded by repeat testing, then the cause of the hyponatremia should be determined based on history, physical exam, urine osmolality, serum osmolality, urine, sodium and chloride. An assessment of volume status should determine if the patient is volume contracted, normal volume, or volume expanded.

B. Classification Hyponatremic Patients Based on Urine Osmolality

1. **Low urine osmolality (50-180 mOsm/L)** indicates primary excessive water intake (psychogenic water drinking).

2. **High Urine Osmolality (urine osmolality >serum osmolality)**

   a. **High urine sodium (>40 mEq/L) and volume contraction** indicates a renal source of sodium and fluid loss (excessive diuretic use, salt-wasting nephropathy, Addison's disease, osmotic diuresis).

   b. **High urine sodium (>40 mEq/L) and normal volume** is most likely caused by water retention due to a drug effect, hypothyroidism, or the syndrome of inappropriate antidiuretic hormone secretion (SIADH). In SIADH, the urine sodium level is usually high, but may be low if the patient is on a salt-restricted diet. SIADH is found in the presence of a malignant tumor or a disorder of the pulmonary or central nervous system.

   c. **Low urine sodium (<20 mEq/L) and volume contraction,** dry mucous membranes, decreased skin turgor, and orthostatic hypotension indicate an extrarenal source of fluid loss (gastrointestinal disease, burns).

   d. **Low urine sodium (<20 mEq/L) and volume-expansion, and edema** is caused by congestive heart failure, cirrhosis with ascites, or nephrotic syndrome. Effective arterial blood volume is decreased. Decreased renal perfusion causes increased reabsorption of water.

III. Treatment of Water Excess Hyponatremia

A. Determine the Volume of Water Excess

   Water excess = total body water x [(140/measured sodium) -1]

B. Treatment of Asymptomatic Hyponatremia. Water intake should be restricted to 1,000 mL/day. Food alone in the diet contains this much water, so no liquids should be consumed. If an intravenous solution is needed, an isotonic solution of 0.9% sodium chloride (normal saline) should be used. Dextrose should not be used in the infusion because the dextrose is metabolized into water.

C. Treatment of Symptomatic Hyponatremia

1. If neurologic symptoms of hyponatremia are present, the serum sodium level should be corrected with hypertonic saline. Excessively

rapid correction of sodium may result in a syndrome of central pontine demyelination.

2. The serum sodium should be raised at a rate of 1 mEq/L per hour. If hyponatremia has been chronic, the rate should be limited to 0.5 mEq/L per hour. The goal of initial therapy is a serum sodium of 125-130 mEq/L, then water restriction should be continued until the level normalizes. The plasma sodium should be raised by no more than 8 mm/dL during the first 24 hours.

3. The amount of hypertonic saline needed is estimated using the following formula:
Sodium needed (mEq) = 0.6 x wt in kg x (desired sodium - measured sodium)

4. Hypertonic 3% sodium chloride contains 513 mEq/L of sodium. The calculated volume required should be administered over the period required to raise the serum sodium level at a rate of 0.5-1 mEq/L per hour.

5. Concomitant administration of furosemide may be required to lessen the risk of fluid overload, especially in the elderly.

IV. Hypernatremia

A. Clinical Manifestations of Hypernatremia

1. Signs of either volume overload or volume depletion may be prominent.

2. Clinical manifestations include tremulousness, irritability, ataxia, spasticity, mental confusion, seizures, and coma. Symptoms are more likely to occur with acute increases in plasma sodium.

B. Causes of Hypernatremia

1. Net sodium gain or net water loss will cause hypernatremia

2. Failure to replace obligate water losses may cause hypernatremia, as in patients unable to obtain water because of an altered mental status or severe debilitating disease.

3. Diabetes Insipidus: If urine volume is high but urine osmolality is low, diabetes insipidus is the most likely cause.

V. Management of Hypernatremia

A. Acute treatment of hypovolemic hypernatremia depends on the degree of volume depletion.

1. If there is evidence of hemodynamic compromise (eg, orthostatic hypotension, marked oliguria), fluid deficits should be corrected initially with isotonic saline.

2. Once hemodynamic stability is achieved, the remaining free water deficit should be corrected with 5% dextrose water or 0.45% NaCl.

3. The water deficit can be estimated using the following formula:
Water deficit = 0.6 x wt in kg x [1 - (140/measured sodium)]

B. The change in sodium concentration should not exceed 1 mEq/liter/hour. Roughly one half of the calculated water deficit can be administered in the first 24 hours, followed by correction of the remaining deficit over the next 1-2 days. The serum sodium concentration and ECF volume status should be evaluated every 6 hours. Excessively rapid correction of hypernatremia may lead to lethargy and seizures secondary to cerebral edema.

C. Maintenance fluid needs from ongoing renal and insensible losses must also be provided. If the patient is conscious and able to drink, water should be given orally or by nasogastric tube.

VI. Mixed Disorders
  A. **Water excess and saline deficit** occurs when severe vomiting and diarrhea occur in a patient who is given only water. Clinical signs of volume contraction and a low serum sodium are present. Saline deficit is replaced and free water intake restricted until the serum sodium level has normalized.
  B. **Water and saline excess** often occurs with heart failure, edema and a low serum sodium. An increase in the extracellular fluid volume, as evidenced by edema, is a saline excess. A marked excess of free water expands the extracellular fluid volume, causing apparent hyponatremia. However, the important derangement in edema is an excess of sodium. Sodium and water restriction and use of diuretics (furosemide) are usually indicated in addition to treatment of the underlying disorder.
  C. **Water and saline deficit** is frequently caused by vomiting and high fever and is characterized by signs of volume contraction and an elevated serum sodium. Saline and free water should be replaced in addition to maintenance amounts of water. §

Hypercalcemic Crisis

Hypercalcemic crisis is defined as an elevation in serum calcium that is associated with volume depletion, mental status changes, and potentially life-threatening cardiac arrhythmias. Hypercalcemic crisis is most commonly caused by malignancy-associated bone resorption. A hypercalcemic crisis occurs when the increased calcium load from the destruction of bone overwhelms the capacity of the kidney to excrete calcium.

I. Diagnosis
  A. Hypercalcemic crisis is often complicated by nausea, vomiting, hypovolemia, mental status changes, and hypotension.
  B. A correction for the low albumin level must be made because ionized calcium is the physiologically important form of calcium.

  Corrected serum calcium (mg/dL) = serum calcium + 0.8 x (4.0 - albumin [g/dL])

  C. Most patients in hypercalcemic crisis have a corrected serum calcium level greater than 13 mg/dL.
  D. A short QT interval suggests the presence of hypercalcemia. Bradyarrhythmias, heart blocks, and cardiac arrest may also occur.

II. Treatment of hypercalcemic crisis
  A. Normal saline should be administered at 2 to 4 L/day until the patient is normovolemic. If signs of fluid overload develop, furosemide (Lasix) can be given to promote sodium and calcium diuresis. Thiazide diuretics, vitamin D supplements, and antacids containing sodium bicarbonate should be discontinued.
  B. Pamidronate disodium (Aredia) is the agent of choice for long-term treatment of hypercalcemia. A single dose of 90-mg infused IV over 24 hours should normalize calcium levels in 4 to 7 days. The pamidronate dose of 30-90 mg IV infusion may be repeated 7 days after the initial dose. Smaller doses (30 or 60 mg IV over 4 hours) are given every few weeks to maintain normal calcium levels. An elevation in temperature

may occur after pamidronate; therefore, acetaminophen should be given before the infusion.

C. Calcitonin (Calcimar, Miacalcin) has the advantage of decreasing serum calcium levels within hours; 4 to 8 U/kg SQ/IM q12h. Calcitonin used alone usually does not normalize serum calcium levels. Therefore, calcitonin should be used in conjunction with pamidronate in severely hypercalcemic patients.

Hypophosphatemia

I. **Clinical Manifestations:** Heart failure, muscle weakness, tremor, ataxia, seizures, coma, respiratory failure, delayed weaning from ventilator, hemolysis, rhabdomyolysis.

II. **Differential Diagnosis of Hypophosphatemia**
   A. Increased Urinary Excretion: Hyperparathyroidism, renal tubular defects, diuretics.
   B. Decrease in GI absorption: Malnutrition, malabsorption, phosphate binding minerals (aluminum-containing antacids).
   C. Abnormal Vitamin D Metabolism: Vitamin D deficiency, familial hypophosphatemia, tumor-associated hypercalcemia.
   D. Intracellular Shifts of Phosphate: Diabetic ketoacidosis, respiratory alkalosis, alcohol withdrawal, recovery phase of starvation.

III. **Labs:** Phosphate, SMA 12, LDH, magnesium, Cal, albumin, PTH, urine electrolytes. 24h urine phosphate, and creatinine.

IV. **Diagnostic Approach to Hypophosphatemia**
   A. **24 hr Urine Phosphate:**
      1. If 24 hour urine phosphate is less than 100 mg/day, the causes include gastrointestinal losses (emesis, diarrhea, NG suction, phosphate binders), vitamin D deficit, refeeding, recovery from burns, alkalosis, alcoholism, DKA.
      2. If 24 hour urine phosphate is greater than 100 mg/day, the causes include renal losses, hyperparathyroidism, hypomagnesemia, hypokalemia, acidosis, diuresis, renal tubular defects, and vitamin D deficiency.

V. **Treatment**
   A. **Mild Hypophosphatemia (1.0-2.5 mEq/dL)**
      1. Na or K phosphate 0.25 mMol/kg IV infusion at the rate of 10 mMoles/hr (in NS or D5W 150-250 mL), may repeat as needed.
      2. Neutral phosphate (Nutra-Phos), 2 capsules PO bid-tid (250 mg elemental phosphorus/tab, 7 mEq Na+ & 7 mEq K+/tab) **OR**
      3. Phospho-Soda (129 mg phosphorus, 4.8 mEq Na+/mL) 5 mL PO bid-tid.

B. **Severe Hypophosphatemia (<1.0 mEq/dL)**
1. Na or K phosphate 0.5 m Moles/Kg IV infusion at the rate of 10 mMoles/hr (NS or D5W 150-250 mL), may repeat as needed.
2. Add potassium phosphate to IV solution in place of KCl (max 80 mEq/L infused at 100-150 mL/h). Max IV dose 7.5 mg phosphorus/kg/6-8h **OR** 2.5-5 mg elemental phosphorus/kg IV over 6-8h. Give as potassium or sodium phosphate (93 mg phosphate/mL and 4 mEq Na+ or K+/mL). Do not mix calcium and phosphorus in same IV.

Hyperphosphatemia

I. **Clinical Manifestations of Hyperphosphatemia:** Hypotension, bradycardia, arrhythmias, bronchospasm, apnea, laryngeal spasm, tetany, seizures, weakness, psychosis, confusion.
II. **Clinical Evaluation of Hyperphosphatemia.**
   A. **Exogenous Phosphate Administration:** Enemas, laxatives, diphosphonates, vitamin D excess.
   B. **Endocrine Disturbances:** Hypoparathyroidism (hypocalcemia will often cause hyperphosphatemia), acromegaly, PTH resistance.
   C. **Rule Out Excess Phosphate Production:** Rhabdomyolysis, sepsis, fulminant hepatic failure, severe hypothermia, hemolysis, acidosis, renal failure, chemotherapy, tumor lysis syndrome.
   D. **Labs:** Phosphate, SMA 12, Cal, parathyroid hormone. 24h urine phosphate, creatinine.
III. **Therapy:** Correct hypocalcemia, restrict dietary phosphate, saline diuresis.
   A. **Moderate Hyperphosphatemia:**
   1. Aluminum hydroxide (Amphojel) 5-10 mL or 1-2 tablets PO ac tid; aluminum containing agents bind to intestinal phosphate, and decreases absorption **OR**
   2. Aluminum carbonate (Basaljel) 5-10 mL or 1-2 tablets PO ac tid **OR**
   3. Calcium carbonate (Oscal) (250 or 500 mg elemental calcium/tab) 1-2 gm elemental calcium PO ac tid. Keep calcium-phosphate product <70; start only if phosphate <5.5.
   B. **Severe Hyperphosphatemia:**
   1. Volume expansion with 0.9% saline 1 L over 1h if the patient is not azotemic.
   2. Dialysis is recommended for patients with renal failure.

References
Al-Shamadi SM, Cameron EC, Sutton RA, AW. J. Kidney Dis 1994; 24:737-52
De Marchi S, Cecchin E, Banile A, Bertotti A: NEJM 1993; 329: 1927-34
Berger W, Keller U: Treatment of diabetic ketoacidosis and non-ketotic hyperosmolar diabetic coma. Baillieres Clin Endo and Metab, Jan, 6(1):1, 1992.
Cefalu WT: Diabetic ketoacidosis. Critical Care Clinics, Jan7(1):89, 1991.
Israel RS: Diabetic ketoacidosis. Emerg Med Clin of North Am, Nov, 74):859, 1989.

Commonly Used Formulas

A-a gradient = $[(P_B - PH_2O) FiO_2 - PCO_2/R] - PO_2$ arterial

$= (713 \times FiO_2 - pCO_2/0.8) - pO_2$ arterial

$P_B = 760$ mmHg; $PH_2O = 47$ mmHg; $R \approx 0.8$
normal Aa gradient <10-15 mmHg (room air)

Arterial O2 content = $1.36(Hgb)(SaO_2) + 0.003(PaO_2)$

O2 delivery = CO x arterial O_2 content

Cardiac output = HR x stroke volume
Normal CO = 4-6 L/min

$SVR = \dfrac{MAP-CVP}{CO_{L/min}} \times 80 = $ NL 800-1200 dyne/sec/cm^2

$PVR = \dfrac{PA-PCWP}{CO_{L/min}} \times 80 = $ NL 45-120 dyne/sec/cm^2

Normal creatinine clearance = 100-125 mL/min(males), 85-105(females)

Body water deficit (L) = $\dfrac{0.6(\text{weight kg})([\text{measured serum Na}]-140)}{140}$

Osmolality mOsm/kg = $2[Na+ K] + \dfrac{BUN}{2.8} + \dfrac{glucose}{18} = $ NL 270-290 $\dfrac{mOsm}{kg}$

Fractional excreted Na = $\dfrac{U Na/ \text{Serum Na} \times 100}{U Cr/ \text{Serum Cr}} = $ NL<1%

Anion Gap = Na + K-(Cl + HCO3)

For each 100 mg/dL ↑ in glucose, Na+ ↓ by 1.6 mEq/L.

Corrected
serum Ca$^+$ (mg/dL) = measured Ca mg/dL + 0.8 x (4-albumin g/dL)

Basal energy expenditure (BEE):
Males=66 + (13.7 x actual weight Kg) + (5 x height cm)-(6.8 x age)
Females= 655+(9.6 x actual weight Kg)+(1.7 x height cm)-(4.7 x age)

Nitrogen Balance = Gm protein intake/6.25-urine urea nitrogen-(3-4
gm/d insensible loss)

Commonly Used Drug Levels

Drug	Therapeutic Range*
Amikacin	Peak 25-30; trough <10 mcg/mL
Amiodarone	1.0-3.0 mcg/mL
Amitriptyline	100-250 ng/mL
Carbamazepine	4-10 mcg/mL
Chloramphenicol	Peak 10-15; trough <5 mcg/mL
Desipramine	150-300 ng/mL
Digoxin	0.8-2.0 ng/mL
Disopyramide	2-5 mcg/mL
Doxepin	75-200 ng/mL
Flecainide	0.2-1.0 mcg/mL
Gentamicin	Peak 6.0-8.0; trough <2.0 mcg/mL

Imipramine	150-300 ng/mL
Lidocaine	2-5 mcg/mL
Lithium	0.5-1.4 mEq/L
Nortriptyline	50-150 ng/mL
Phenobarbital	10-30 mEq/mL
Phenytoin**	8-20 mcg/mL
Procainamide	4.0-8.0 mcg/mL
Quinidine	2.5-5.0 mcg/mL
Salicylate	15-25 mg/dL
Theophylline	8-20 mcg/mL
Valproic acid	50-100 mcg/mL
Vancomycin	Peak 30-40; trough <10 mcg/mL

* The therapeutic range of some drugs may vary depending on the reference lab used.
** Therapeutic range of phenytoin is 4-10 mcg/mL in presence of significant azotemia and/or hypoalbuminemia.

Index